1,001
Home
Remedies

Tips & Tricks for Natural Health & Beauty

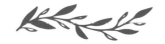

Mary Rose Quigg

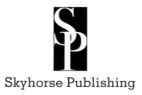

Skyhorse Publishing

Skyhorse Publishing books may be purchased in bulk at special discounts for sales promotion, corporate gifts, fund-raising, or educational purposes. Special editions can also be created to specifications. For details, contact the Special Sales Department, Skyhorse Publishing, 307 West 36th Street, 11th Floor, New York, NY 10018 or info@skyhorsepublishing.com.

Skyhorse® and Skyhorse Publishing® are registered trademarks of Skyhorse Publishing, Inc.®, a Delaware corporation.

Visit our website at www.skyhorsepublishing.com.

10 9 8 7 6 5 4 3 2 1

Library of Congress Cataloging-in-Publication Data is available on file.

Cover design by David Ter-Avanesyan
Cover images by Shutterstock

Print ISBN: 978-1-5107-6226-8
Ebook ISBN: 978-1-5107-7041-6

Printed in China

Contents

Acknowledgments

I would like to dedicate this book to my family for all the encouragement they give me. A special word of thanks to my friend Martina for her assistance with the research and to Mena for promoting my books.

Introduction

*"To ensure good health: Eat lightly, breathe deeply,
live moderately, cultivate cheerfulness,
and maintain an interest in life."*
—William Londen

This collection of hints is an invaluable guide to modern wellness. Many of the hints are the product of tradition passed from one generation to another.

Natural products, available at local stores or found in your kitchen, are used in many of the potions and beauty aids.

The hints cover advice on care of the body from head to toe, beauty treatments, habit control, a common sense approach to first aid and using medicines.

I've enjoyed compiling this practical, informative book and I hope you find something of interest to help improve the quality of your daily life.

—Mary Rose

A MEDICINAL DRINK

"Take a cup of caring,
And two large spoonfuls of kindness.
Mix well with a dash of sympathy,
Blended with a little firmness.
Add a splash of humour and gaiety,
Together with plenty of patience.
Dose the patient frequently and
add a cuddle if necessary to
aid a speedy recovery."

The Medicine Chest

First Aid Box

A clearly labeled first aid box should contain:

- Adhesive bandages
- Antacid medicine
- Antiseptic ointment
- Antiseptic solution
- Antiseptic throat lozenges
- Aspirin
- Bandages (an assortment)
- Burn wipes or spray
- Calamine lotion
- Cotton balls
- Cough syrup
- Deep heat rub
- Gauze
- Kaopectate or Pepto-Bismol
- Laxatives
- Safety pins
- Scissors
- Soothing eye lotion

The locked medicine cupboard should have:

- Travel sickness tablets
- Tylenol tablets/liquid
- Vapor rub

• • • •

For an emergency, keep the name and telephone number
of the local doctor and hospital in your first aid kit
or clearly posted in your home.

• • • •

Useful information regarding members of the household should include past illnesses and subsequent treatment, as well as dates of previous operations or stays in hospital. Note any allergies or long-term medication. Include details of immunizations.

. . . .

At least once a year, take everything out of the medicine cabinet and check expiration dates. Dispose of all outdated medicine. If uncertain about any product, call a pharmacist and ask what the shelf life is.

. . . .

Always store medicines in their original containers. Some medicines come in tinted glass, because exposure to light may cause them to deteriorate.

. . . .

Discard old hardened or cracked tubes of cream. Dispose of any liquid medicines that appear cloudy or filmy.

. . . .

Every medication is a potential poison. Keep all medicines and vitamins locked in a high cabinet, well out of children's reach.

. . . .

Do not try to diagnose a health problem yourself and do not stop taking prescribed medication or commence taking complementary treatments without consulting your doctor.

. . . .

To make insect repellent, combine 10 drops essential oil (basil, eucalyptus, cloves, geranium, peppermint, rosemary, lemon balm (citronella), onions, garlic, and/or feverfew) and 2 tablespoons vegetable oil in a glass jar; stir to blend. Dab a few drops on your skin or clothing. Pregnant women should consult with their doctor before using essential oils.

. . . .

When stung by an insect, first remove any remaining stinger with a pair of tweezers. Avoid squeezing the poison sac as this pushes the remaining poison into the skin.

. . . .

For bee and ant stings, apply a solution of baking soda and water, while for wasp stings use vinegar. Dry the area and cover with a cold compress.

. . . .

If stung in the mouth, suck an ice cube or rinse out the mouth with a solution of cold water and baking soda. Watch out for swelling, which can cause breathing difficulties.

. . . .

A severe allergic reaction to a sting will result in a state of shock; in this case get medical help as soon as possible.

. . . .

Chamomile flower tea relieves a headache.

. . . .

To soothe a sty, grate a carrot finely and put into a piece of muslin or a fine cotton handkerchief. Dab on the sty frequently until it comes to a head.

. . . .

Use cayenne pepper to treat cuts or minor wounds. It will sting, but it helps to stop the bleeding.

. . . .

For a sore throat, add 1 teaspoon of cider vinegar to a glass of water and gargle. Alternatively, gargle with a glass of water containing 1 teaspoon (5 milliliters) each of salt and baking soda or chew a piece of raw onion.

. . . .

For mouth ulcers, peel a clove of garlic and cut off a slice. Place the cut end on a mouth ulcer and squeeze the juice onto it.

. . . .

For corns, crush a garlic clove and put onto the corn. Cover with an adhesive bandage. Renew daily.

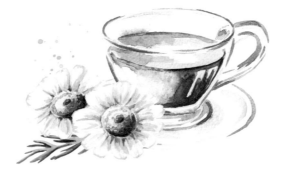

Ginger tea can be gargled to ease a sore throat, or sip it to quell motion sickness.

. . . .

Honey is a natural healer for cuts, burns, or chapped lips.

. . . .

Apply an ice pack to sprains and bruises for fast relief. Use cubes or crushed ice in a strong plastic bag and wrap in a towel or cloth. Only use the ice pack for 10 minutes at a time. Never use an ice pack on blisters or wounds, if the patient has circulatory problems, or is hypersensitive to cold.

. . . .

For constipation, before breakfast every day, drink a glass of warm water with a little lemon juice added.

. . . .

To soothe a headache, cut a lime in half and rub it on your forehead.

. . . .

For chilblains, rub twice daily with a slice of onion dipped in salt.

. . . .

To relieve toothache, soak a piece of cotton in clove or garlic oil and pack next to the painful tooth.

. . . .

Chew sprigs of parsley to remove the smell of garlic from the breath or to relieve flatulence.

. . . .

Tincture of cayenne can be rubbed on painful gums.

. . . .

To get rid of itch from mosquito bite, apply soap on the area for instant relief.

. . . .

Put scotch tape over a splinter, then pull it off to remove the splinter painlessly and easily.

. . . .

Thyme and tea tree oil will clean a wound and stop infection but will also sting.

. . . .

Speedy immersion in cold water for at least 10 minutes is essential for minor burns. Then treat with a mixture of 1 part lemon juice or vinegar and 3 parts water. Apply to the affected area with cotton balls.

. . . .

Other remedies for minor burns are milk of magnesia, a paste of baking soda and water, or golden syrup. Always get medical attention for severe burns.

. . . .

Dip a cotton swab in vanilla extract and apply to a painful tooth and surrounding gum area.

. . . .

"When wealth is lost, nothing is lost; when health is lost, something is lost; when character is lost, all is lost."
—Billy Graham

To relieve itchy skin or sunburn, add 3–4 tablespoons vinegar to a warm bath and soak in it for 10 minutes.

. . . .

For cold sores, mix 5 milliliters vodka with 2 drops each of tea-tree, bergamot, and eucalyptus oils. Dab on the sore often during the day to stop a blister forming.

HOME REMEDIES

When using prescribed medicines or when pregnant, do not use any herbal remedies without first consulting your doctor.

. . . .

Asthma: Combine ¼ cup onion juice, 1 tablespoon honey, and ½ teaspoon black pepper. Take 1 teaspoon regularly.

. . . .

Arthritis: Drink parsley tea made by pouring a cupful of boiling water over 1 teaspoon chopped parsley. Let it infuse until cool, strain, and sip throughout the day.

. . . .

Baby colic: Crush 1 teaspoon caraway, dill, or fennel seeds, and soak in 1 cup (250 milliliters) boiling water for ½ hour. Strain and use 1 teaspoon of the liquid when necessary.

. . . .

Bad breath: Put ½ tablespoon ground cinnamon, 1 tablespoon ground cloves, and 1 tablespoon ground nutmeg into a bowl, and mix well. Stir in ¼ pint (150 milliliters) sweet sherry, pour into an airtight bottle, and leave for 3 days. Strain and rebottle. Add a few drops to a glass of water to rinse the mouth. Or simmer ¼ cup vinegar, ½ cup wine, ¼ cup honey, and 1 teaspoon ground cloves. Add to cold water and use as a mouthwash.

. . . .

To ward off bladder infections, drink ½ cup of cranberry juice daily.

. . . .

Bloating: Before breakfast, take 1 teaspoon cider vinegar and 1–2 teaspoons honey in a glass of warm water.

. . . .

Boils: To draw out boils, make a poultice of bread soaked in hot milk between two layers of clean, fine cotton. Place over the affected area and keep in place with a cotton bandage. An onion peeled and baked until soft can also be used.

. . . .

Bruises: Rub a little to a liberal amount of butter on a bruise. Or eat fresh pineapple or drink pineapple juice.

. . . .

Burns in the kitchen, sunburns, and chemical burns: Spread mustard very generously to burned area and let dry. If pain persists, rinse with cold water and re-apply mustard. Or spread egg white on a burn and let dry—it feels cool and removes the sting from the burn as it dries.

. . . .

Chapped lips: Mix 5 tablespoons almond oil with 1 tablespoon melted beeswax. Rub on as required to soothe.

. . . .

Chest congestion: Add some peppermint essence or friar's balsam to a bowl of boiling water. Drape a towel over your head and lean over the bowl, staying at least 9 inches (22 centimeters) above the water. Inhale the steam for about 5 minutes. This will loosen any mucus in the nose or throat and help you breathe more easily. Do not use this treatment on sensitive skin.

. . . .

Cold prevention: Put 4 pints (2.2 liters) hot water into a basin, and add 1 heaped teaspoon dried mustard. Soak feet for 10 minutes before going to bed.

. . . .

Also for cold prevention, at bedtime, steep 1 tablespoon elderflower in a cup of boiling water for 20 minutes. Strain, add honey to taste, and drink hot.

. . . .

Cold sores: When first signs of a cold sore appears, apply witch hazel with a cotton swab. It will immediately stop the process, and prevent further spread of blisters. Apply frequently to encourage healing.

. . . .

Press a wet tea bag against a cold sore to act as an antiseptic. The tannin from the tea will help reduce the condition.

. . . .

"Imagination is not a talent of some men but is the health of every man."
—Ralph Waldo Emerson

As soon as the tingling of a cold sore starts, take 2 Brewer's Yeast pills; this will shorten its duration.

. . . .

Common cold: Using a heat-resistant glass, add 1–2 peeled and crushed cloves of garlic, ½ grated rind and all the juice of 1 lemon, a pinch of cayenne pepper, ½ teaspoon ground ginger, and 1 tablespoon honey. Stir well to mix and add a ½ pint (300 milliliters) of nearly boiling water. Allow to cool, and drink the whole lot, including the solids. After taking this concoction go straight to bed and stay there until you feel fit and well again.

. . . .

Reduce the length of a cold from weeks to days by not blowing your nose. Just wipe the nostril gently with a paper tissue when it starts to run.

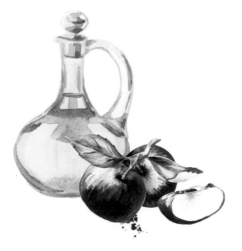

To relieve coughs:
- Add 5 cloves of peeled and crushed garlic to 8 ounces (225 grams) honey. Cover and let stand for 24 hours. Take 1 teaspoon of the resulting juice hourly.
- Make a garlic syrup: Put 9 ounces (250 grams) crushed garlic in a 1¾ pint (1 liter) jar. Fill with equal amounts of water and cider vinegar. Cover and leave for a few days, and stir occasionally. Strain and add 1 cup honey and refrigerate. Take 1 tablespoon three times a day.
- Boil 2 young turnips until soft, purée with a little of the cooking water, and add a little milk and 2 teaspoons honey. Eat often.
- Mix 1 teaspoon turmeric powder in a glass of lukewarm milk, add sugar if needed, and take it before bedtime.
- To relieve a troublesome nightly cough, add 1 teaspoon black treacle or molasses and a pinch of nutmeg to a glass of hot milk and drink before going to bed.
- To expel phlegm, draw the air in through the nose, then cough with good force.
- For a dry irritating cough, to $\frac{1}{3}$ pint (200 milliliters) boiling water, add the juice of 1 lemon, 2 teaspoons honey, ¼ teaspoon cinnamon, 1 clove garlic, and a sprig of rosemary. Stir well, cover, and leave for 15 minutes. Strain and sip slowly.

· · · ·

Cramps: Cramps are the stiffening of the muscles into a spasm, usually after exertion, caused by a buildup of acid in the muscles. For relief from cramps, dip a towel in hot water and place it over the affected area. Massage a mixture of ½ olive oil and ½ clove oil into the muscle. Eat a banana daily.

· · · ·

Cystitis: At the first signs of an attack of cystitis, drink a glass of water with 1 teaspoon of baking soda added, every hour for 3 hours.

. . . .

For another cystitis remedy, pour ½ pint (300 milliliters) of boiling water over 1 teaspoon powdered marshmallow root. Stir and leave for 20 minutes. Add 1 teaspoon honey, and take the whole mixture 3 times a day before meals.

. . . .

Dehydration: If you do not drink enough fluids during the day, the body runs the risk of becoming dehydrated. At least 4 pints (2 liters) water should be drunk daily. Symptoms of dehydration can be taut skin, dry mouth, muscle cramp, dark urine, constipation, thirst, lethargy, sunken eyes, and headaches.

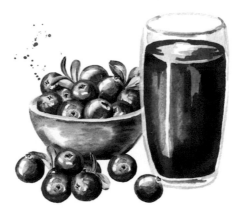

"The cure for anything is salt water—sweat, tears, or the sea."
—Isak Dinesen

Diaper rash:
- Soak 1 teaspoon dried or 2 teaspoons fresh elderflowers in 1 pint 600 milliliters boiling water. Cover and leave for 20 minutes. When cool, apply to the affected area with sterile gauze.
- Boil ⅛ teaspoon boric acid in 4 pints (2.4 liters) water. Cool, soak a cloth, and apply to baby's bottom, then leave on as long as possible. Wipe off and sprinkle on cornstarch. Or make a paste of cornstarch and water and apply when changing the diaper.

. . . .

Diarrhea:
- Eat well-cooked, salted rice and drink the water it was cooked in or eat a grated apple that has been left to go brown. Drink plenty of liquid.
- Cover 2 ounces (50 grams) pearl barley with cold water, simmer for 2 minutes, and strain. Place the barley, 2–3 teaspoons sugar, thinly pared rind of half a lemon, and 1 pint (600 milliliters) boiling water in a jug. Cover and strain when cold. Use to replenish lost fluid or mix with ready-made rehydration medication sachets to make them more palatable.

. . . .

Earache:
- Slice an onion in half and put it over the ear hole for ½ hour at a time or until the pain subsides.
- Chop a clove of garlic and simmer in ¼ cup of oil for 20–30 minutes. Strain carefully and cool. Use slightly warm as ear-drops in the morning and at bedtime. Plug ears with cotton for 10 minutes.

. . . .

Eczema: Steep ½ ounce (13 grams) chamomile flowers in 1 pint (600 milliliters) boiling water for 20 minutes and add to a bath for relief.

. . . .

Flatulence: Drink a mug of hot milk with a cinnamon stick in it or sprinkle 1 teaspoon cinnamon on top, or eat a dill pickle and 1 teaspoon of the pickling liquid.

. . . .

Fungal infections:
- Soak 10 nettle stems with leaves in 4 pints (2.2 liters) cold water for 1 hour. Heat until hot to the touch, then strain. Use to bathe infected hands or feet, for ½ hour daily.
- Half fill 1 pint (600 milliliters) bottle with finely chopped and washed nettle roots. Add a little alcohol and cork tightly. Leave for three weeks. Paint on this solution as required.

. . . .

Gout: Drink 3–4 cups of yarrow, dandelion, or celery seed tea every day or simmer 3 corn cobs in 4 cups (1 liter) of water. Strain and refrigerate. Heat and drink after meals.

- Eat 4 ounces (100 grams) fresh cherries daily.
- Apply a leek poultice to the part affected.
- Elevate the joint and take ibuprofen. Never take aspirin for gout.
- Apply ice and drink lots of water.
- Do not eat anchovies, gravy, sardines, cauliflower, mushrooms, clams, oatmeal, shellfish, spinach, and do not drink alcohol.

. . . .

Hay fever: Three to four months before the hay fever season, start taking 1 tablespoon natural honeycomb 3 times a day.

· · · ·

Headache: Eat 10–12 almonds instead of two aspirin for a migraine headache. Almonds rarely upset the stomach. To ease a migraine, sit with the feet in a bowl of cool water.

· · · ·

Combine ¼ cup almond oil, 20 drops rosemary oil, 20 drops lavender oil, and 30 drops of peppermint oil. Mix thoroughly and gently massage temples and forehead with the mixture. Place a small amount near your nostrils and inhale this relaxing scent. This should bring relief for most headaches. If the pain persists, massage the back of your neck and fleshy area between your thumb and index finger as well.

· · · ·

Place a bag of frozen peas or crushed ice between the neck and the head on the side that the pain mainly occurs. This will help relax the neck muscles and constrict the nerves.

· · · ·

When a headache threatens, apply firm pressure with the thumb on the web between the other thumb and index finger for 2 minutes. Repeat on the other hand. Pregnant women should not use this massage.

· · · ·

For a sinus headache, place equal parts of natural apple cider vinegar and water in a small pan over heat and allow to boil slowly. When the fumes begin to rise from the pan, lean your head over it until the fumes are comfortably strong. Inhale for 50–80 breaths to alleviate the headache.

. . . .

Hiccups:
- Chew fresh mint leaves. Make a drink with 2 teaspoons crushed dill seeds in a little hot water, infuse for a few minutes, strain, and dilute with cold water before drinking.
- Lick 1 tablespoon peanut butter off a spoon or take 1 teaspoon sugar, honey, or marmalade and let it slowly melt on your tongue.
- While drinking a glass of water with a straw, plug your ears with your fingers, or take a glass of water, tilt your head upside down, and drink out of the glass.
- Just take 7 sips of any fluid or drink a glass of water, then eat a piece of bread.
- Put your hands above your head and stretch for a few minutes, or pull the top of your hair for 1–2 minutes.
- Open your mouth as wide as you can. Put a cotton swab far back in the roof of your mouth and gently rub.
- Suck a wedge of a lime or drink ½ shot glass of lemon juice; a little sugar can be added to make it more palatable.
- Take a deep breath and say the word "purple" slowly as you breathe out.

. . . .

Nausea and travel sickness: Infuse ½ teaspoon grated ginger root in a cup of boiling water for a few minutes, strain, and drink.

• • • •

Nettle stings: Rub the affected area with the liquid from the base of a dock leaf or with a slice of onion.

• • • •

Perspiration:
• For deodorant powder, put ½ cup baking soda, ½ cup cornstarch, and a few drops essential oils such as lavender or cinnamon in a glass jar, and shake to blend. Sprinkle a light covering of the powder on a damp cloth. Pat on. Do not rinse.
• For a liquid deodorant, combine ¼ cup each witch hazel extract, aloe vera gel, and mineral water, 1 teaspoon vegetable glycerin, and a few drops antibacterial essential oils such as lavender (optional) in a spray bottle. Shake to blend.

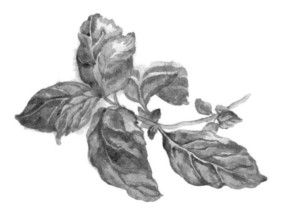

Throat: To ease a sore throat, try eating one finely chopped onion mixed with honey. Or combine the juice of ½ lemon and 1 cup of glycerin and sip regularly.

. . . .

Scars: Break open a vitamin E gel capsule and apply a generous amount of the oil to a scar. Takes about one month to remove a recent scar, but longer for older ones.

Sinus blockage: Onion is a natural decongestant. Slice an onion and cover with 1–2 tablespoons sugar, and leave for ½ hour until juice forms. Take 1 teaspoon juice hourly.

. . . .

Sprained ankle: Apply a hot lettuce or cabbage poultice to prevent a sprained ankle swelling up.

. . . .

Stomach upset: Simmer 1 teaspoon cinnamon and honey in water for 20 minutes, cool, and sip slowly. For an acid stomach, make meadowsweet tea and sip after meals.

. . . .

Stys: Put a raw egg in a white cloth and place on eye for 15 minutes, 3 times a day to help draw out a sty.

. . . .

Tiredness or fatigue: Pour ½ pint (300 milliliters) of boiling water over 1 teaspoon rosemary leaves, infuse for 30 minutes, strain. Drink ½ cup warm infusion first thing in the morning and at bedtime.

. . . .

Tonic: Infuse a handful of dandelion leaves in boiling water for 10 minutes. Strain and drink 3 cups daily.

. . . .

Rosehip syrup: Cover 4 pounds (1.8 kilograms) rosehips with water and bring to the boil. Simmer until soft. Put the pulp into a muslin bag and squeeze out the juice and reserve. Return the pulp to the pan and repeat the process. Add all the juice to a clean muslin bag and allow to drip into a basin. Add 2 pounds (900 grams) sugar to the juice, stir, and boil for 5 minutes. Bottle and seal immediately. Take 1 teaspoon daily as a tonic during the winter months.

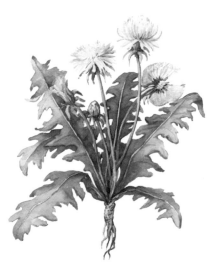

Thrush: Put a handful of marigold leaves into boiling water, and leave for 10 minutes. Remove the leaves from the liquid and add 2 drops lavender oil. Bathe the affected area with the cooled solution. Plain yogurt can also relieve itching.

· · · ·

Tongue burn: To soothe a burnt tongue, sprinkle a little sugar on the tip.

· · · ·

Toothache:
- Soak a cotton ball in the juice of a grated raw onion and press onto the affected tooth.
- Chew on a clove of garlic while waiting to go to the dentist. After tooth extraction, use an infusion of lady's mantle or chamomile flowers to rinse out the mouth and as a gargle.

· · · ·

Whooping cough: Add 1 tablespoon chopped thyme leaves to 1 pint (500 milliliters) water. Bring to the boil, remove from the heat, and infuse for 10 minutes. Drink the strained liquid regularly.

· · · ·

Warts: Pour ¼ pint (150 milliliters) boiling water over 2 ounces (50 grams) of ivy leaves. Cool and strain. Dampen a cotton ball with the ivy water, apply to the wart, and cover with an adhesive bandage twice daily. Slowly the wart will soften and fall off.

Eyes, Ears, Nose, Mouth & Brain

THE EYES HAVE IT

People with blue eyes are more prone to cataracts. Pigment melanin protects the eye by trapping light rays. Pale-colored eyes contain less melanin in the iris than dark colored eyes. This leaves them more sensitive to direct sunlight and more prone to macular damage in the form of cataracts or loss of vision.

• • • • •

To help prevent eye problems, it is sensible to eat dark green vegetables and orange-yellow vegetables that are rich in carotenoids and citrus and kiwi fruits, rich in vitamin C.

• • • • •

Vitamin E found in nuts, seeds, and oily fish is a preventative, while bilberry aids normal vision and maintains healthy eye tissue and blood flow.

• • • • •

No matter what size, color, or shape eyes are, if they are bright and sparkling they look beautiful. When happy the eyes dance and shine, while if tired, bored, or miserable the eyes will be dull and listless.

• • • • •

Puffy eyes can be due to lack of sleep, too much sleep, sensitivity to certain products, using too rich a moisturizer on the delicate skin around the eyes, poor circulation, or a possible thyroid problem or constipation.

• • • • •

Dark circles can be due to lack of sleep, exercise, or fresh air, poor circulation, possible kidney problems, food intolerance, or nutritional deficiencies.

. . . .

Tired eyes can be due to reading or writing in poor light, lack of sleep, or working on a computer for too long a period.

. . . .

Droopy eyes can be due to age and lack of muscle tone.

. . . .

Wrinkled eyelids can be due to age, exposure to irritants, sluggish circulation, or diet.

. . . .

Crow's feet can be due to age, dehydration, sun damage, or facial expressions like squinting.

. . . .

Our eyes are one of our most beautiful and individual features, but they need care to look their best. Remove signs of tension around the eyes by massage. Begin near the nose, taking the eyebrows between the finger and thumb and moving outwards towards the temples, pinching lightly.

. . . .

To refresh your eyes, lie down for 10 minutes with your feet 1 foot (30 centimeters) above the head, and with thighs and legs supported by cushions. Cover the eyes with cucumber, cold tea bags, or cotton wool pads soaked in witch hazel, chamomile, rosehip, or fennel tea.

• • • •

Use chilled segments of melon to soothe eye puffiness.

• • • •

To soothe puffy eyes, spoon 1 tablespoon aloe gel into a small jar, add 15 drops jojoba oil, 15 drops evening primrose oil, 1 capsule vitamin E oil, and 2 drops rose essential oil. Stir well to blend. Smooth over the eyes and relax for 10 minutes. This mixture will keep chilled for up to four weeks.

• • • •

To revive tired eyes, place fresh apple peel (do not use if gone brown) or soak used black tea bags in cold water for 10 minutes and place them on the puffy area. Leave on the eyes and rest for 10 minutes.

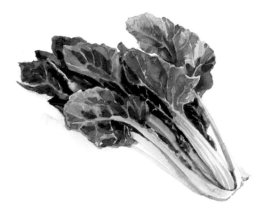

Hold a metal spoon under cold running water for a few minutes and then gently press it onto the eye area for at least a minute to soothe, cool, and reduce swelling. Or cover eyes with thin cucumber slices.

. . . .

Place thin slices of raw potato underneath your eyes. The potassium in them counteracts dark circles.

. . . .

For an eye cream, melt 1 tablespoon lanolin in a heat-proof bowl over a pan of hot water, and add 1½ tablespoons almond oil. Remove from the heat and slowly add 1 teaspoon powdered lecithin, beating constantly. Add 2 teaspoons cold water and mix well.

. . . .

To restore luster to eyes, infuse 4 tablespoons fresh eyebright or 2 tablespoons dried herb in 2 cups hot water. Leave to cool, strain, and bottle. Bathe the eyes regularly with the mixture.

Eye Exercises

For taut eyelids, shut both lids tightly for 15 seconds, then rest the eyes by keeping them lightly closed. Repeat 5 times.

. . . .

To strengthen muscles, keeping the head still, move the eyes as far to the right as possible without straining, blink, then do the same to the left. Blink and repeat 6 times on each side. Lightly close the eyes and rest for a minute.

. . . .

*"Obstacles are those frightful things you see
when you take your eyes from your goal."
—Henry Ford*

Keeping the head still, raise the eyes as high as you can, blink once, then lower the eyes as far you can. Blink again and repeat the exercise 6 times. Rest.

· · · ·

Keeping the head still, look up towards the right eyebrow, blink, and look down towards the left earlobe. Repeat 6 times, rest for a minute. Repeat, looking towards the left brow and the right lobe.

To improve eyesight, first thing every morning and last thing at night, splash the closed eyes 20 times with warm water and then 20 times with cold to stimulate circulation.

· · · ·

Keeping the body stationary, slowly move the eyes and head from side to side, through 180 degrees, so the open eyes trace a smooth arc without fixing or glazing over. At the end of each arc, check the eyes are still pointing in the same direction as the nose. For more effect do this exercise outside on a sunny day, with the eyes closed and the sunlight on the eyelids. Then do the following palming exercise: Sit comfortably with the eyes closed and elbows resting on a table. Gently place slightly cupped palms over the eyes to block out light, leaving the nose free. Do not apply any pressure to the eyeball. Breathe deeply, relax, and concentrate on the darkness or listen to soothing music for at least 10 minutes, three times a day.

· · · ·

Remember to blink frequently, once or twice every 10 seconds, when concentrating hard. If the eyes feel gritty then blink rapidly a few times. This is especially needed if wearing contact lenses. Do not stare at objects; move gaze from one point to another.

. . . .

Rest the eyes periodically by looking into the distance; the farther away you look the more relaxation is given to the eye muscle.

. . . .

Hold two pencils or the index fingers in front of the face, one about 3 inches (8 centimeters) away, the other at arm's length. Focus on one with both eyes, blink, then focus on the other.

EYE PROBLEMS

For many people, the eye area is a real problem. This is one of the first areas to show the signs of ageing and is also a problem area for fluid retention. Elevate the head when you sleep to encourage fluid to drain away from the eye area.

. . . .

Certain moisturizers can cause the eye area to swell up. Use special eye creams or gels if you have puffy or ageing eyes.

. . . .

Avoid salty foods as these can cause fluid retention.

. . . .

Stys are caused by a bacterial infection on the edge of the eyelid, within one of the oil-secreting glands. They are usually caused by the staphylococcus bacterium. Generally the infection will be gone in 3-4 days, though a persistent stye will need to be drained by a qualified doctor.

• • • •

Recurring stys are usually a sign of a vitamin A deficiency. Loss of eyelashes can often accompany this problem and taking vitamin B will help prevent this.

• • • •

Bathing the eye in lukewarm wash of raspberry leaf tea can help prevent infections and reduce inflammation when a sty occurs. Never squeeze or puncture a sty as this worsens the infection.

• • • •

A foreign body in the eye is one of the most common emergencies. The tiniest speck of dirt, metal, or grit can cause an immense amount of discomfort and irritation. When this occurs, do not rub the eye. Sit the person on a chair facing the light. Stand behind the chair and let the head rest against you. Separate the lids of the affected eye and look for the foreign body. If it is in a very obvious position, remove with the dampened corner of a clean handkerchief, gauze, or a moistened cotton swab. It also can be flushed out with clean warm water or saline solution. Or bathe the eye with warm milk to remove the object and the gritty feeling. Sometimes blowing the nose moves a speck to the inner corner of the eye making it easier to remove. If it is under the upper lid, grasp the lashes and pull the lid down over the lower lid. Do not poke the eye with any instruments. When there is difficulty in removing the object, cover the eye with a clean pad, secure lightly, and get medical help.

• • • •

To test for satisfactory eyesight, you should be able to read a car's license plate number at an 80-foot (23-meter) distance.

· · · ·

Eyesight should be checked regularly. Frowning to see or read something in the distance is a nuisance and can causes wrinkles.

· · · ·

Good quality sunglasses should be worn in bright sunshine, especially when driving.

· · · ·

To check the quality of lens in sunglasses, hold them at arm's length. Look through each lens separately at a slim vertical object. Rotate the lens slightly; the vertical image should remain true if the lens is of good quality.

· · · ·

Wear protective goggles when travelling on a motorcycle, welding, working power tools, or in a dusty environment.

· · · ·

Since tears contain a high proportion of stress chemicals, most people generally feel better after crying.

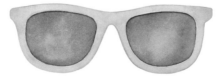

When symptoms of redness, itching, and swollen eyelids develop, it is probably an allergy to cosmetics. Remove all make-up until the symptoms disappear. Do not use the product again.

. . . .

Do not borrow or lend eye cosmetics, as infections are easily passed from person to person.

. . . .

It is advisable to buy eye make-up from a reputable manufacturer.

. . . .

Avoid putting on eye make-up when travelling as the eye can be accidentally poked with the brush or pencil.

. . . .

People with contact lenses usually require special make-up to avoid irritation.

. . . .

Always apply and remove mascara gently to avoid pulling out eyelashes.

. . . .

Remove all eye make-up before going to bed.

. . . .

When doing close-up work, make sure there is adequate lighting. Flickering lights should be repaired immediately.

. . . .

Natural lighting is best, but if a lamp is used, then position it so that the light comes over the shoulder. An adjustable desk lamp will give a softer light than an overhead fluorescent one.

EARS & NOSE

Small glands in the outer ear canal are constantly producing wax to protect the sensitive lining of the ear from infection, and this soft wax is continually being brushed out by tiny hairs. Sometimes this wax becomes hard and blocks the outer ear, causing deafness.

. . . .

Do not attempt to clean the wax out with cotton swabs as you could push it into the ear canal and cause damage to the eardrum. Instead, put a few drops of warm olive oil into the ear twice a week and the wax may soften and extract itself. A doctor can remove the wax by syringing or remove any small hard lumps of wax with a probe.

. . . .

Wax or tweeze ear hairs, but if you want to cut them, ask someone to help you.

It is not true that ears adjust and become accustomed to noise. Any problems due to damage of the middle or outer ear are irreparable. The level of noise should be reduced or leave the source if it causes your ears to hurt or ring, you have to shout to be heard, or you feel slightly deaf after the noise has stopped.

. . . .

Always wear special ear protectors when using power tools or in a noisy workplace. Buy a good quality personal stereo to ensure good reception with less volume. Never wear headphones for longer than an hour at any given time.

· · · ·

Limit time at rock concerts or clubs to two hours. Cover the ears to muffle the sound of planes taking off or when a subway train pulls in to the station. Avoid buying children noisy toys or ones with explosive sounds.

· · · ·

If exposed to a high degree of constant noise, have periodic hearing checks. Always be aware that noise is not just irritating, it can also be a danger to your health.

· · · ·

When there is pain or ringing in the ear, a discharge, or you suspect that there may be a foreign body lodged inside, consult a doctor as soon as possible.

· · · ·

For earache, crush a clove of garlic into olive oil. Leave for 10 minutes and strain. Slightly warm the oil and pour into the ear. Do not use this treatment if the eardrum could be perforated and do not repeat if the ear remains painful.

· · · ·

Do not be tempted to purchase a hearing aid without having a proper examination by your doctor.

· · · ·

Nosebleeds

Nosebleeds, or epistaxis, can be quite alarming. The lining membrane of the nose has a rich supply of tiny veins and if these are damaged, they bleed profusely.

· · · ·

Young children often have nosebleeds due to picking their nose. Soften any scabs or crusts inside the nose with petroleum jelly or, if there is infection, ask your doctor to prescribe an antibiotic cream.

· · · ·

Children with allergies are more prone to nosebleeds as they tend to sneeze and blow their nose more frequently.

· · · ·

Before trying to stop a nosebleed, give the nose a good blow to remove any clot that may be holding open a broken blood vessel.

· · · ·

To stop a nosebleed, sit the person on a chair with their head slightly bent over a bowl or sink. With the thumb and forefinger, firmly pinch the lower part of the nostril together. Hold for 10–15 minutes. Breathe through the mouth. Slowly release the nostrils. If the bleeding continues, pinch for a further 10 minutes.

· · · ·

To stop a nosebleed, dip a cotton swab in witch hazel or rosewater and dab on the inside of the nostril.

· · · ·

If bad breath isn't due to anything serious, use better oral hygiene to remove the problem. Brush the teeth more frequently and floss teeth after meals to clean spaces your toothbrush can't reach.

. . . .

Gently brush tongue to rid the surface of a stagnant coating of bacteria or food that can build up and give off unpleasant odors. Use rosewater or a strong infusion of mint as a mouthwash.

. . . .

Visit the dentist to have teeth professionally cleaned every six months. Stop smoking.

. . . .

There are about 3,000 taste buds on the tongue, palate, back of the mouth, throat, and tonsils. These buds can detect four sensations: sweet and salt at the tip of the tongue, acidity or sour at the sides, and bitterness at the back.

. . . .

Look at the tongue regularly in daylight before brushing the teeth to get a measure of your general health

. . . .

Look at the tongue in sections. The front represents the chest, the mid-section the abdomen, and the solar plexus (part of the nervous system behind the stomach) and the back section covers the lower abdomen and lumbar region.

. . . .

Observation of the tongue will not tell you what exactly is wrong but can be a useful way to know if you need to seek medical expertise.

. . . .

The normal tongue is pinkish-red, moist with a slight shine, a uniform flat shape, and has no thick coating, spots, or lines.

. . . .

A red tongue could be due to inflammation or dehydration in the specific area. Drink at least 8 glasses of water a day.

. . . .

A very pale tongue shows a blood deficiency or a lack of energy, perhaps due to a lack of iron or certain vitamins. Take a daily multivitamin and mineral supplement and eat plenty of fresh fruit and vegetables.

. . . .

A blue tinged tongue may be due to circulatory problems, an excess of sugar, chemicals including medication, or processed foods including juices, soft drinks, and alcohol.

The coatings of the tongue arise from various toxins that are present in the body.

. . . .

A white coating can be due to phlegm or toxins caused by an excess intake of "cold" foods such as dairy products or wheat. Cut down on these foodstuffs.

. . . .

"Believe a quarter of what you hear, half of what you see, and three-quarters of what you know."
—Unknown

A yellow coating can be due to phlegm or toxins due to an excess intake of "hot" food such as curries, sugar, alcohol, or coffee. Cut down on these foods and drinks.

. . . .

A gray tongue can be due to a phlegm accumulation from a cold or flu virus. Cut down on dairy products.

. . . .

Peeled patches on the tongue indicate a moisture deficiency in the specific area.

. . . .

A swelling at the tip of the tongue can point to heart problems. When other areas of the tongue are swollen this indicates too much fluid accumulating in the relevant part of the body. Drink more fluids.

. . . .

Cracking and dryness of the tongue generally indicates dehydration. Cracking at the center of the tongue suggests digestive problems. Adjust your diet and drink more fluids. Cracks at the tip can be due to emotional or stress-related problems. Cracks at the sides are due to poor food and fluid metabolism. Eat more slowly and take more exercise. Fine cracks to the left of the front portion of the tongue are a sign of smoking, giving rise to breathing problems.

. . . .

A tooth-marked or scalloped edged tongue suggests congestion of the lymphatic system.

. . . .

A very moist tongue, especially with a thick, greasy coating, may indicate excess fluids in the body, possibly due to a build up of mucous. Flat spots along the sides suggest emotional frustration. Try a calming therapy. Raised white spots on the root of the tongue show an accumulation of toxins in the abdomen. Consider a detox day of fresh fruit and vegetables only, once a week. Red points on the tip indicate anxiety and stress. Deep-breathing exercises may help. Purple-colored spots show a sluggish bowel flow.

. . . .

To relax the tongue, place it behind your front teeth.

. . . .

The chief cause of tooth decay is plaque; this is a rough sticky substance made up of saliva, bacteria, and food debris.

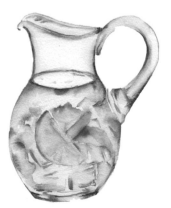

Plaque forms almost continuously around the teeth and gums; unless it is removed by regular brushing and flossing, it will eat away at the tooth enamel and cause cavities.

· · · · ·

A build-up of plaque hardens into a deposit on the teeth called tartar; this can be felt with the tongue. Only a dentist or dental hygienist can remove plaque successfully.

· · · · ·

Bacteria in plaque use the sugar in food to form acid that erodes the tooth's enamel. Acidity can last up to 2 hours after a meal so the number of meals consumed is as relevant as the food eaten.

· · · · ·

Limit sweet foods to mealtimes and at the end of a meal have a small piece of cheese as this helps neutralize the acid.

· · · · ·

Avoid eating late at night as the saliva flow decreases when we sleep and the mouth will not be properly cleansed.

· · · · ·

Saliva neutralizes acid in the mouth. People who suffer from a dry mouth may find it beneficial to chew sugar-free gum for a minimum of 20 minutes after a meal.

DENTAL CARE

Brush the teeth regularly for 2–3 minutes, especially after breakfast and at bedtime, with fluoride toothpaste. Brush the upper teeth downwards and the lower teeth upwards, to stop pushing the gums away from the teeth. Pay attention to all biting surfaces. Hold the toothbrush in a pen-like grip to avoid excessive force.

. . . .

Replace a toothbrush when the head starts to lose its shape or at least every three months. Dentists recommend that a toothbrush should have medium to soft nylon bristles, a flat even brushing surface, densely packed bristles, a straight handle, and a medium to small head rounded at the end.

. . . .

Dental floss can dislodge trapped food and remove plaque from crevices in the teeth. Floss is available as waxed or unwaxed and as dental tape that is wider and easier to use.

. . . .

To use dental floss, take 2 feet (60 centimeters) of floss and wrap the ends around the middle fingers until you have around 3 inches (7.5 centimeters) to work with. Hold the floss taut between the thumbs or index fingers to guide it between the teeth. Rub on both sides of each tooth, using a new section of floss each time.

. . . .

Stop smoking as it stains the teeth. Have a dental check-up every six months.

. . . .

Clean teeth by mixing 2 tablespoons fine sea salt with 3 tablespoons baking soda, store in a dry airtight non-metal container. To use, shake a little of the mixture into your hand and pick it up with a damp toothbrush.

. . . .

Most mouthwashes do more harm than good, as they contain alcohol, which dries out the mucus membranes and gum linings, which make them more prone to infection. Instead, rinse the mouth with a glass of warm salty water.

. . . .

If gums tend to bleed, rinse the mouth with a solution of salt and water. Report bleeding gums or any other problems to the dentist during regular check-ups.

. . . .

To preserve a tooth knocked out in an accident, do not clean the tooth; use disinfectant on it or let it become dry. The best method is to immediately immerse the tooth in a cup of whole milk where it will keep for up to twelve hours, allowing time to visit the dentist to have it reinserted in the socket. It is important, however, to have the tooth replaced in the socket as quickly as possible. The nerve endings tend to die and the socket begins to heal, causing the reinsertion to be unsuccessful.

BRAIN POWER

Most of us use only a small portion of our available brain power. We should not limit our abilities but learn to use our whole brain.

. . . .

The brain is divided into four quadrants, each with particular skills and functions. The left frontal tends to be logical, analytical, and used for making decisions. The left back is tuned into fine detail and used to follow instructions. The right front generates creative, visual, and imaginative ideas. The right back is closely connected to our emotions.

· · · ·

To develop logic, analytic thought, and critical faculties:
· Predict 10 events, however small, about tomorrow, based on things that have happened.
· Learn how the washing machine works, or how to program your DVR to record a show.
· List five weaknesses in a favorite novel, film, or play.
· Learn to play bridge, chess, or another game that's new to you.

· · · ·

To stimulate the imagination:
· Take a long walk or leisurely drive, without feeling guilty.
· Invent a new "gourmet" dish or a whole meal.
· Imagine what your life will be like in 5–10 years' time.
· Close your eyes and create a beautiful daydream; don't reproach yourself for wasting time.

· · · ·

To develop discipline and attention to detail:
· Assemble a model kit, following the instructions carefully.
· Arrange books in alphabetical order.
· Work out what you are worth in monetary terms by adding up all the money you have in financial institutions.
· Draw up a personal budget.
· Organize the garden shed, the attic, or your desk.
· Be on time for appointments for a week.

· · · ·

"Ability is what you're capable of doing.
Motivation determines what you do.
Attitude determines how well you do it."
—Lou Holtz

To develop emotions and intuition:
- Play with children but let them take the lead.
- With your eyes closed, imagine yourself dancing but without moving your body.
- Take 10 minutes every morning to imagine how each member of your family is feeling at that moment.
- Pick up a pebble or flower and absorb its beauty.
- Watch a sad film and let the tears flow.
- Lose yourself in your favorite piece of music.

IMPROVING THE MEMORY

Difficulty in remembering names can be overcome by using picture association. When introduced to someone called Charlie, imagine him with a bowler hat and a moustache like Charlie Chaplin or link the person's name to a feature of their face.

· · · ·

To remember numbers, associate each number with a letter, 1=a, 2=b, 3=c, up to 9=i. 0 can be o or j. Make a word or phrase from each number. If your bank pin number is 1528 (AEBH), make the phrase An Eternal Big Headache.

· · · ·

If you have trouble remembering where you parked the car, take a few minutes to imprint the image of your car in your head; include a nearby landmark, such as a building.

· · · ·

Exercise regularly. Aerobic exercise like jogging, brisk walking, or swimming increases the circulation to the brain.

. . . .

Nourish the brain with breathing exercises. Inhale deeply, then exhale for twice as long. Do this a few times to increase the oxygen to the brain.

. . . .

A good night's sleep will help the brain function more effectively.

. . . .

The left side of the brain is used for logic, the right side for imagination. To improve the way they work together, draw a large figure 8 horizontally, in the air or on paper, with each hand 8 times, and then with both hands together 8 times. Or march slowly for 5 minutes, lifting the knees quite high. As each knee is raised, touch it with the elbow of the opposite arm. Do these two exercises regularly.

. . . .

Make lists of things you need to remember. The mere act of writing them down will fix it in your mind. Rewrite the list from memory and compare the two.

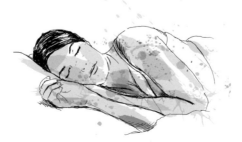

Hair Health

FACTS ABOUT HAIR

Physiologically, the hair is dead—only the root is growing—but it can be a barometer of your general state of health.

. . . .

All hairs on the body are produced from small nodules (papilla) at the base of follicles (small indentations) in the skin, which are connected to a blood supply.

. . . .

In the scalp, the size of the follicle dictates the thickness of the hair while its shape determines whether the hair is straight, wavy, or curly.

. . . .

Hair mainly comprises of a protein called keratin. It has a life-span of between a few months to several years before falling out, depending on diet and treatment of the hair.

. . . .

Follicles rest for up to six months before producing a new hair. There are 100,000–150,000 hair follicles on the head.

. . . .

Every day between 50 and 150 hairs are lost. Hair grows at the rate of about a ½ inch (1 centimeter) per month, a little faster in warm weather.

The maximum length of hair is normally 3 feet (90 centimeters) but there are exceptions to this with one recorded case of hair growing to 10 feet (3 meters) long.

. . . .

Eyelashes are the only hairs on the body that do not turn gray with age. There are around 200 lashes on each eye.

. . . .

Dry hair can either be because your glands are under-active, or you've damaged your hair with chemical treatments, heated appliances, harsh handling, or overexposure to the sun. Often, curly hair is dry as the natural oil tends to stay at the root instead of working its way down the hair length.

. . . .

Fine hair is more likely to be greasy because there is less hair to soak up the sebum. Hormonal imbalances speed up oil production, as can poor diet, stress, over handling, and even cold weather.

. . . .

Combination hair is greasy at the roots and dry at the ends. The longer your hair is, the more it becomes dry and brittle due to harsh treatment, while the roots stay greasy.

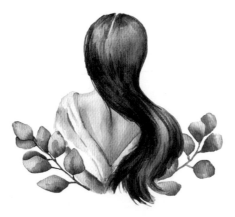

A biotin rich drink of bananas blended with honey, yogurt, and low-fat milk can help regenerate hair follicles, but does not cure any underlying conditions or stress-related hair loss.

HEALTHY HAIR

The developing hair in the follicle gets nourishment from food eaten, so a good diet is essential for healthy hair.

. . . .

Dry hair has split ends, is of rough texture, and can be frizzy. Over use of hair dryers, heated gadgets, bleaching, and UV rays all leech moisture from the hair shaft, exposing the central core to the elements. Blocked hair follicles that prevent the natural oils from moisturizing the hair shaft can also be a cause of dry hair.

. . . .

Minimize the use of heated gadgets, do not use the hottest setting, and stop while the hair is still slightly damp. Avoid styling products containing isopropyl or ethyl. Gently brush the hair from root to tip to help distribute the oil in the hair. Use conditioning treatments.

. . . .

Apply hair conditioner before soaking in the bath; the heat helps the conditioner absorb into the hair follicles.

. . . .

When using wax, gel, or serum, less is more. Only apply a small amount of chosen product. Applying too much to the front, especially, will make the hair look greasy.

. . . .

Serum is best for creating a smooth glossy finish while wax is used to define and separate the hair. Do not use wax on long thick hair or it will make it look greasy and tangled.

· · · ·

Hair suffers from a lot of wear and tear resulting in split ends. Many products claim to repair split ends but the best remedy is a regular trim by a reputable stylist.

· · · ·

To have healthy hair, the scalp must be firm and supple. Poor circulation to the scalp is the cause of many hair problems. Good blood flow and lymphatic circulation to and from the scalp prevents toxic build-up. Massaging the scalp will help circulation and give nourishment to the hair follicles.

· · · ·

For a good scalp massage, dip a cotton wool ball in warm coconut, almond, or olive oil and squeeze out any excess. Apply the oil along the central parting. Continue to part the hair at regular intervals across the front and back of the head applying the oil until the scalp is covered. Replenish the oil on the cotton wool as required. Use the balls of the fingers to manipulate the scalp. Move the scalp, not the fingers. Apply comfortable pressure. At the base of the skull, circle the thumbs along the hairline with the fingers resting on the back of the head. Run the fingers through the hair to disperse the oil. Wrap the head in a plastic shower cap and a warm towel and relax for 10–30 minutes. Wash as normal with warm water.

· · · ·

Brittle hair can be caused by illness, or by some prescribed medicines. It can look smooth and soft but can break easily.

. . . .

Dull hair is mostly due to product overload. Occasionally use a detoxifying shampoo to remove product build-up.

. . . .

Flakiness without itching or oiliness is the symptom of real dandruff.

. . . .

Dandruff can also be caused by seborrhoeic dermatitis that produces an itchy scaly rash on the scalp, eyebrows, beard, chest, back, or groin. Everyone has a small quantity of yeast on the skin but people with dandruff have a large amount.

. . . .

For mild dandruff, shampoo regularly with a gentle anti-dandruff shampoo. For more severe problems, use shampoos containing coal tar, pyrithione, selenium, sulphide, or anti-fungal agents such as ketoconazole. These products reduce flaking and help to control the excess yeast cells present. There is a wide range of shampoos available containing these products and only by trial and error will you find the one that best suits your problem.

. . . .

Use special treatment shampoos only while the problem persists, as they dry out the hair. If over-the-counter treatments do not clear up the problem in a couple of weeks it may be necessary to consult a doctor to avail of stronger products available by prescription.

. . . .

Wet hair with beer before setting with rollers. Or add volume to limp hair by giving the hair a final rinse with beer diluted in warm water, after shampooing and conditioning.

. . . .

It is important to wash the hair properly. With a wide toothed comb or a bristle brush, comb or brush the hair to remove tangles and any surface dirt before washing.

. . . .

To avoid splitting hair, start combing the ends first and work your way upward. Do not start at the roots.

. . . .

Avoid brushing or combing hair too frequently during the day as this creates static and can cause the hair to split.

. . . .

To avoid static from hairbrushes, keep them squeaky clean by washing with a drop of shampoo and warm water. Or sprinkle some baking soda directly onto the brush or comb and then spray with vinegar. This will create a foaming reaction. Leave for 5 or 10 minutes and rinse clean.

. . . .

Never wash the hair in bath water; use a shower attachment.

. . . .

A rich creamy shampoo is best for hair that has been chemically treated with a perm or color.

. . . .

Thoroughly wash and rinse hair as soon as possible after swimming. If salt water dries on hair, it can cause mineral deposits to build up.

. . . .

There are many homemade shampoos for every type of hair and you will find some of these included in this book, starting on page 61.

. . . .

To wash hair, first soak with warm water to wet the hair thoroughly. Put a small blob of shampoo on the palms of the hands and smooth it over the hair gently. Massage the shampoo into the scalp and down to the ends of the hair. Do not rub.

. . . .

If your hair is long, only lather the scalp—the rest will be washed with the soapy water as you rinse. Rinse thoroughly until the water runs clear.

. . . .

Unless the hair is very dirty, one shampoo wash is sufficient.

. . . .

A lot of lather means the product is high in detergent and extra care must be taken to make sure it is all rinsed out.

. . . .

Avoid tangles by letting the hair fall straight and naturally. Wet hair is weaker and more easily damaged than dry, so treat gently.

. . . .

Dry hair and scalp should be rinsed in very warm water to stimulate oil production. With oily hair, cool water is recommended.

. . . .

All hair types appreciate a conditioning rinse; normal and fine hair will benefit from a weekly treatment, while dry and chemically treated hair will need an application after every shampoo.

. . . .

After washing hair, blot dry with a towel and then gently comb conditioner through the hair. Leave for a few minutes before rinsing thoroughly.

. . . .

Choose the conditioner to suit your type of hair. Conditioner may only need to be used 2-3 times a week.

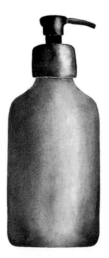

Shampoo basically strips the hair of grime and natural oils while conditioner lubricates. Since they work in totally different ways, shampoo and conditioner combined products should only be used occasionally.

. . . .

Intensive conditioning treatments can be given to hair about once a month. These are designed to penetrate deeper than ordinary conditioners and are not rinsed out after applying.

. . . .

If using a body-building gel or mousse to give volume to lifeless hair, do not use it on wet hair as it will make the hair go limp. Water will dilute the active ingredients in the gel or mousse. Instead, towel dry hair to remove excess moisture, then massage the gel or mousse into hair and style as usual.

. . . .

Use mousse or gels sparingly as they can cause build-up that will dull hair and weigh it down.

. . . .

Hair can stretch up to a third of its length when wet but returns to normal when dry. However, if hair is wrapped around tight rollers or small brushes when blow-drying, this can make the hair brittle.

. . . .

Do not keep hair tied back tightly constantly as this can lead to thinning around the hairline.

. . . .

Where possible, let the hair dry naturally, but not in the sun as the wet hair absorbs the ultraviolet rays and can damage the hair. Turn your head upside down and use your hands to shape and lift the roots for volume.

. . . .

Consult a hairdressing salon for products to use on problem hair.

. . . .

When feeling unwell and unable to wash greasy hair, warm a clean towel and rub the hair vigorously with it for a few minutes. It will look freshly groomed.

. . . .

Keep the hair covered in very hot, cold, or windy weather.

NATURAL HAIR CARE

Here are several home remedies for dandruff:
- Mix 1 part antiseptic mouthwash with 9 parts water, pour over the scalp, and massage in. Leave for 5–10 minutes and rinse well.
- Add 2 teaspoons cider vinegar to two beaten egg yolks, wet the hair, and massage in the egg mixture. Leave for 10 minutes and then rinse.
- Pour ¼ pint (150 milliliters) boiling water over 4 tablespoons dried rosemary and leave to infuse for an hour. Strain and add 2 tablespoons each of olive oil and castor oil. Massage into the wet hair and leave for 10 minutes. Rinse well.
- Dissolve 3 aspirin in 50 milliliters normal shampoo and use to wash hair.
- Blend 2 tablespoons olive oil, lemon juice, and mineral water and apply to the scalp. Leave for 15 minutes and shampoo as usual.

- Add 1 teaspoon each of lavender and rosemary to a cup of witch hazel. Leave to infuse for 5 days, then rub the mixture into the scalp every night.

· · · · ·

Aloe Vera gel or the contents of a vitamin E capsule rubbed into the scalp will remove loose dandruff flakes and soothe the scalp.

· · · · ·

Condition the hair and prevent dandruff with a nettle rinse. Wear rubber gloves to cut young nettles. Wash and put in an enamel saucepan. Cover the nettles with cold water, bring to a boil, and simmer for 15 minutes. Strain and allow to cool before use. Add ¼ pint (150 milliliters) cider vinegar to every 1 pint (600 milliliters) nettle water. Massage into the scalp daily.

· · · · ·

As a hair rinse, add 2 tablespoons dried rosemary to 2 pints (1.2 liters) boiling water, bring to a boil, and simmer for 10 minutes. Cool and infuse for 2 hours. Strain and add ¼ pint (150 milliliters) cider vinegar. Bottle and label the mixture. After washing the hair, rinse off the shampoo thoroughly, then pour a few cupfuls of the rosemary infusion over the hair. Towel dry. Or add 2 tablespoons cider vinegar and 1 tablespoon rosewater to 2 pints (1.2 liters) warm water. Use this as a final rinse.

· · · · ·

Revitalize hair dried out from central heating by mixing the contents of a vitamin E capsule and 1 tablespoon wheat-germ oil. Apply to the ends of the hair and comb through with a wide-toothed plastic comb. Cover with a plastic cap and wrap in a warm towel for 15 minutes. Wash thoroughly and allow to dry naturally.

· · · · ·

Things that Matter
It's the little things that matter,
Like a baby's toothless grin,
Or a chat with friends and neighbors
And the words "now do call in."
It's a letter on the doormat
And a cheery cup of tea,
Or an act of simple kindness
That's performed in secrecy.
—Unknown

For shiny hair, add a cup of white vinegar to a jug of hot water. Allow to cool while washing and rinsing the hair. Holding the head over a bowl, pour the mixture over it. Reuse the water a few times, then finally rinse with cool water. Give hair this treatment every two months.

. . . .

To give hair a shine, mash an overripe banana and combine with 3 drops of almond oil. Massage into dry hair and leave on for 15 minutes. Shampoo as usual.

. . . .

To help remove the build-up from products and to give you naturally clean hair, mix 1 teaspoon baking soda in the palm of your hand with your favorite shampoo. Wash as usual and rinse thoroughly.

. . . .

Leave a bottle of beer open overnight, pour into a plastic cup, and heat in the microwave for 10 seconds. Add 2 teaspoons honey. Stir and rinse hair with mixture and leave on for 2 minutes. Repeat twice a week. This is good for color-treated hair. Or rinse hair with cold chamomile tea to clear product residue.

. . . .

Beer and lemon make an effective cleansing shampoo: use 1 lemon and ½ pint (300 milliliters) of brown ale. Squeeze the lemon juice into the beer and apply to damp hair. Massage well, leave for a few minutes, then rinse thoroughly.

. . . .

For a hair tonic, soak 2 ounces (50 grams) nettles, 1 ounce (25 grams) rosemary, and 1 ounce (25 grams) marigold petals in 8 fluid ounces (250 milliliters) vodka for three weeks. Strain and add three drops of lavender essential oil and 4 fluid ounces (100 milliliters) distilled water. Massage into the hair and scalp three times a week.

. . . .

Whisk 1 egg and ¼ pint (150 milliliters) yogurt. Massage into hair after shampooing, and leave for 5 minutes. Rinse off with tepid water.

. . . .

For greasy hair, add ¼ cup lemon juice to ⅓ cup regular shampoo. Wash as usual. This will also add highlights.

. . . .

For limp hair, mix 1 pint (600 milliliters) bitter or mild beer (preferably flat) with ⅛ pint (75 milliliters) cider vinegar. Pour over freshly washed hair and leave to absorb for 5 minutes before toweling dry. The smell disappears once the hair dries.

. . . .

For flyaway hair, mix ½ mashed avocado with 1 tablespoon mayonnaise and apply to newly washed hair. Leave on 10 minutes, then rinse thoroughly. Use once a week.

. . . .

For fine dry hair, beat 1–2 egg yolks with 1 teaspoon mild shampoo. Wet hair with tepid water and shampoo hair with the mixture. Rinse well with tepid water.

. . . .

For very dry hair, whisk 2 tablespoons olive oil, 1 tablespoon cider vinegar, and one egg yolk together until smooth. Massage through damp hair and then cover the head with a plastic shower cap and a warm towel. Leave for 30 minutes and then shampoo off using lukewarm water.

. . . .

To restore luster to parched hair, mix avocado pulp with a little honey and apply before washing.

. . . .

As a conditioning treatment, mix 1 part honey to 3 parts olive oil in a jar, leave for a few hours, and shake well. Massage into the hair, shampoo as usual, and rinse with a mixture of ½ cup cider vinegar and 2 pints (1.2 liters) water.

. . . .

For a quick hair conditioner, using an electric beater, mix 1 egg, 2 tablespoons castor oil, 1 teaspoon cider vinegar, and 1 teaspoon glycerin. Or combine 1 egg with 1 teaspoon honey and 2 teaspoons coconut or olive oil. Massage into the scalp and wrap the head in a plastic cap and a hot towel. Shampoo as usual. Or mix ½ cup brandy, ½ cup water, and 2 egg yolks, beaten. Massage into the hair and leave for 10 minutes. Rinse well with tepid water.

· · · ·

To revive a droopy perm, put 1 teaspoon lime or lemon juice in ½ pint (300 milliliters) cold water and pour over the hair before washing.

· · · ·

For squeaky-clean hair, shampoo hair with 1 teaspoon baking soda mixed into your normal shampoo, and rinse thoroughly. The soda helps remove the build-up from conditioner, mousse, and sprays.

· · · ·

An effective tonic when losing hair is to steep a medium-sized onion cut in slices, in half a cup of rum. Leave for 24 hours. Remove the onion and reserve the liquid. Massage a little amount of the liquid into the scalp every night for a week, then once a week until the hair loss has lessened.

· · · ·

For grey hair, simmer 2 tablespoons dried sage in 1 pint (600 milliliters) water for 10 minutes, cool, and strain. Use as a finishing rinse after every shampoo.

· · · ·

Blonde hair rinse: 2 tablespoons fresh or 1 tablespoon dried chamomile flowers, 2 tablespoons fresh or 1 tablespoon dried marigold flowers, 2 tablespoons fresh lemon juice. Pour 1 pint (600 milliliters) hot water over the flowers and infuse for 30 minutes. Stir in the fresh lemon juice. Strain and use the infusion in the final hair rinse. This mixture will show no effect at first but will gradually lighten the hair over weeks. One of the great advantages is that it does not give a harsh result and leaves the hair soft and smelling lovely.

· · · ·

To bleach fair hair, make an infusion of 4 tablespoons chamomile flowers in a cup of hot water. Leave for 20 minutes. Strain and mix into a paste with kaolin. Apply the paste to the roots of the hair first, then comb through the hair with a wide toothed comb. Leave on for 20–60 minutes, depending on the porosity of the hair and the depth of lighter color required.

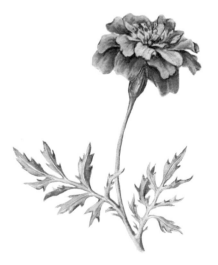

Hair can be lightened with rhubarb dye. Simmer 3 rhubarb roots and stems in 2 cups of white wine or water for 30 minutes. Remove from the heat and leave for 30 minutes. Strain and use the liquid as a rinse or mix with kaolin to make a paste and use as a dye.

. . . .

For lightened hair that has been discolored by chlorine, mix equal amounts of tomato sauce and vodka, apply to the hair, and relax for 15 minutes; shampoo as usual.

. . . .

Dark hair rinse: 2 tablespoons fresh or 1 tablespoon dried sage leaves, 2 tablespoons fresh or 1 tablespoon dried rosemary, 1 pint (600 milliliters) strong tea. Pour the hot tea over the herbs. Leave to infuse for 30 minutes. Strain and use as the final rinse.

. . . .

To highlight brown hair, simmer 2 tablespoons each of dried sage and rosemary in 2 pints (1.2 liters) water for 10 minutes. Leave to infuse for 2 hours. Strain, add ¼ pint (150 milliliters) cider vinegar and bottle. Rinse clean wet hair over a basin; repeat a few times.

. . . .

After shampooing and conditioning brunette or auburn hair, rinse with a cupful of red wine.

. . . .

Enrich hair color naturally: for dark hair, brew one strong cup of espresso; for blond hair, use chamomile tea; and for red hair, use lemon-balm tea. Let cool completely. Pour on dry hair and leave on for 20 minutes. Rinse well.

. . . .

To give light brown hair extra color depth, cover walnut shells with water and bring to a boil. Simmer for 2 hours. Strain off the liquid and store in an airtight, labeled bottle. After washing the hair, apply the liquid to the hair with a pad of cotton wool. Leave for 2 minutes, then rinse off.

. . . .

Henna is a natural dye and rarely causes skin or scalp problems. However, do not use henna if hair has already been colored, tinted, or dyed with a chemical substance, as there can be no guarantee of the finished color.

. . . .

Henna produces different effects on various shades of hair. It can either give the hair highlights or turn it flaming red. Always do a color test on a small strand first. Keep note of the time the dye was left on the hair.

. . . .

Henna can be used to cover gray hair, but only if the percentage of gray is less than 5 percent. Always do a strand test as some henna dyes can give gray hair an orange effect.

. . . .

Make a henna paste with 1 cup henna and 1 cup boiling water or 1 cup henna and 1 cup strong hot tea (brings out more red) or 1 cup henna and 1 cup hot coffee (dulls the red slightly). Heat one of these pastes in a heat-proof bowl over a pan of hot water for 10–30 minutes. Cool, then re-heat to boiling point. Remove from the heat and do a strand test to ascertain the color required. Reheat the mixture until hot enough to apply comfortably. Add 1 beaten egg and 1 tablespoon castor oil. Wearing rubber gloves, apply the hot mixture to the hair. Wrap the head in aluminum foil or plastic cap and wrap in a hot towel. Leave on for required time, judged by the strand test, then wash as usual.

. . . .

To make hair gel to hold unruly hair in place, melt 1 tablespoon castor oil, 1 tablespoon coconut oil, 1 tablespoon petroleum jelly, and 1 teaspoon emulsifying wax in a heat-proof bowl over a pan of hot water. Remove from the heat, add perfume if desired, beat together with an electric beater on a low speed for a few minutes. Leave to cool and use as required.

. . . .

For homemade hairspray, chop 1 lemon (or 1 orange for dry hair) and cover with 2 cups water. Boil until reduced by half. Cool, strain, and place in a spray bottle. Store in the refrigerator. If very sticky, dilute with water or add 2 tablespoons rubbing alcohol as a preservative. The hairspray can be stored for up to 2 weeks unrefrigerated

THE NITTY GRITTY

The most obvious sign of hair lice is frantic scratching of the head, particularly at the back and behind the ears.

. . . .

On close inspection, tiny almost see-through eggs are attached to the hairs, or you might see little dark brown creatures moving through the hair.

. . . .

Lice feed by biting the scalp and sucking the blood. They must be eliminated immediately as they multiply rapidly.

. . . .

The female lays five to eight eggs per night and glues them to the base of the hair, close to the food source. A female louse can lay 50–150 eggs during her one-month lifetime. The youth and adult lice feed on your head several times a day.

. . . .

To get rid of hair lice use an insecticidal or herbal treatment. Follow the instructions on the product carefully. It may be necessary to treat all members of the family. Alert the school or playgroup to let other parents know that their children may need treatment.

. . . .

A natural remedy for head lice: 25 drops rosemary oil, 25 drops lavender oil, 13 drops geranium or pelargonium oil, 75 milliliters almond oil, and 12 drops eucalyptus. Mix the oils together thoroughly. Divide the hair into small sections and saturate each section with the mixture. Leave on for 2 hours. Shampoo to remove, rinse well, and comb through with a fine comb. Repeat after 3 days.

. . . .

Another remedy is to mix 20 drops tea tree oil, 10 drops eucalyptus, and 10 drops rosemary with 2 fluid ounces (60 milliliters) carrier oil such as sweet almond. Apply to the hair and leave overnight. In the morning, wash it out and comb the hair with a fine comb. Following this treatment wash the hair using any shampoo with a few drops of tea tree oil added to it.

Care of the Body

Fitness & Exercise

Fitness is having flexibility, stamina, and strength.

• • • •

Flexibility is being able to comfortably bend, twist, and stretch through a range of movements. When supple you are less likely to get injured and remain more active as you age.

• • • •

Stamina is being able to run or walk briskly without getting tired and out of breath quickly. Good stamina deters heart disease.

• • • •

Strength is being able to exert force for lifting, pulling, or pushing. It is necessary for daily living and protects the body from strains and sprains. A strong core (back, abdominal area, and pelvis area) helps to give good posture.

• • • •

If you are overweight, pregnant, or suffer from back pain or any other medical condition, always consult your doctor before attempting any form of exercise.

• • • •

If you have a cold, sore throat, or a high temperature, do not exercise until you feel better and then start again gradually.

• • • •

Do not do any vigorous exercise for at least 1 hour after a meal. Stop exercising if you feel sick or unwell, in pain, dizzy, or have unusual fatigue.

• • • •

Sometimes an underactive thyroid gland (hypothyroidism) can cause someone to gain excessive weight. Symptoms include lack of energy, increased weight, dry skin, brittle hair, feeling the cold, thickening of ankles and legs, and a slow pulse. If you are worried that you have this problem, seek medical advice.

. . . .

Our body size and structure reflects not only our eating and exercise habits but also our genetics. We are all born with a certain body type inherited from our parents. Although no one is a pure body type, there are three different applicable categories: ectomorphs, mesomorphs, and endomorphs. Most people are a mixture of body types.

. . . .

Ectomorphs have a light build with slight muscular development. They are usually tall and thin with small frames and narrow hips and shoulders.

. . . .

Mesomorphs have a medium frame and muscular build. They often have broad shoulders, and their weight is concentrated in the upper body, making them look compact or stocky.

. . . .

Endomorphs have a heavy, rounded build with shoulders usually narrower than their hips. They have a round, soft appearance and are more often overweight or obese.

. . . .

When we understand and appreciate our bodies, we are able to work with them, not against them. Everyone can improve their health and performance levels by implementing the principles of a safe and effective eating and exercise program.

. . . . .

To lose fat through exercise alone, aerobics is the best method. An aerobic workout must constantly raise the heartbeat and breathing rate for a period of 20 minutes. To start burning fat, the workout should be 30 minutes. Aerobic exercise includes brisk walking, jogging, swimming, and dancing.

. . . . .

Fat burning exercises should be fairly moderate and comfortable. If exercise hurts, you are pushing yourself too hard. Remember, as you become more fit you will have to work harder in order to reach the same level of intensity to burn fat.

. . . . .

Regular exercise is better than sporadic sessions. Start off gently and build up slowly to avoid risks of sprains and strains.

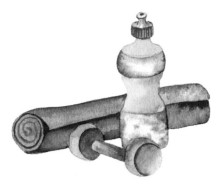

Always warm up first with a few gentle bends and stretches. Cool down after an aerobic exercise session by walking slowly for a few minutes.

. . . .

Exercise should be done regularly 2-3 times a week with no more than 2 days of rest in between. Increase the duration of each session to 1 hour as fitness improves. Keep exercises varied to relieve boredom and prevent the body becoming accustomed to exercise.

. . . .

At the end of an exercise class, to get the whole benefit from it, lie on the floor and stretch out. Relax, close the eyes, and do some good breathing.

. . . .

As fat is burned almost exclusively by the muscles, the fitter the muscles are, the more fat will be burned. People who exercise regularly have far more fat burning enzymes in their body than people who do no exercise.

. . . .

Swimming and cycling give a constant rhythmic heart and lung workout without too much strain on the lower body muscles.

. . . .

When exercising, the body releases hormones called endorphins. These increase the feeling of well-being and help to reduce fat storage.

. . . .

As well as specific exercises, substitute short bus trips with brisk walks. Climb stairs instead of taking the elevator

• • • •

If you have fun while you exercise, it is so much easier to forget you are exercising at all. One way of doing this is to dance, and another way is to go back to childhood games to get back to the basics of fun exercise.

• • • •

Frisbee makes for a good cardiovascular workout as well as toning for the legs, buttocks, and upper body. If partners are not particularly good at throwing, you will have to run around to catch the Frisbee, and you'll have to stretch, too. To add more exercise to the session, build in forfeits for missing the frisbee, like having to do push-ups or sit-ups.

• • • •

Playing tag is a great cardiovascular workout, using lungs and heart, as well as toning the thighs.

• • • •

Hula-Hooping is great for toning the waist. Put the hoop around the waist, hold the arms up, spin the hoop around the waist, and gyrate the hips in a circular motion to keep the hoop up.

• • • •

Hopscotch is great for toning thighs. In this game, chalk out 1 to 10 on the pavement slabs and jump on the squares, skipping the square the stone lands on. Maximize your upper body workout by using a heavier object that you will have to throw and pick up.

• • • •

Climbing is a good total body workout. It can be done on a climbing frame at a gym, or try rock climbing (with proper equipment and training). You'll need to use the legs to push yourself up, and your arms to pull. Remember, safety first. Always use safety equipment.

. . . .

Twister is great for flexibility and toning upper and lower body. Play with a few partners. In this game you contort into strange shapes; be careful you don't fall and injure yourself.

. . . .

To convert these activities into a full workout, do 10–15 minutes each of tag, frisbee, and hula-hoop.

. . . .

In order for exercise to become second nature, you must find the right motivation. Set yourself some goals and reward yourself. Treat yourself to a manicure or pedicure, a special dinner, or a favorite film.

. . . .

Plot your weekly fitness goals and stick them on the fridge, in the bathroom, and on your mirrors. Pack your bag the night before your gym session and leave it in the car or by the front door.

. . . .

Stand up straight. Weak stomach muscles can cause bad posture. Imagine a string tied to the head pulling you upwards and stretching, straightening the spine. Keep the chin up and head held erect. Push the shoulders gently down and back. The back should be as flat as possible and the stomach comfortably held in. The hips must be tucked in and the knees relaxed.

. . . .

Car controls should be easily reached without stretching. On long journeys, stop frequently to stretch. Move the neck and shoulders when possible to prevent stiffness. Relax, as tension makes the muscles tight and less efficient at absorbing the vibrations from the car. To get out of a car, swing the body sideways before moving the legs out.

. . . .

Before playing tough sports, always warm up.

BEAUTY'S ONLY SKIN DEEP

Skin is designed to be self-cleansing and self-nourishing, but we attack it inwardly with bad diet and outwardly by sun, wind, and pollution exposure and not removing make-up.

. . . .

Care of the skin begins with a healthy diet, high in vitamins, and with combatting stress. Exercise and a proper amount of sleep both play their part.

. . . .

Skin should be cleansed regularly and have sufficient moisture. Skin surface can be covered with flaky dead skin, excreted toxins, and grime. Removing these from the skin and keeping it clean is important for good skin care.

. . . .

Soap and water is an excellent cleanser for the skin. However it is very alkaline and can upset the natural acid balance of the skin. Sometimes this causes dryness and the skin reacts by producing more oil, resulting in greasy skin.

. . . .

Choose soaps that have near the same pH balance as skin or use cream cleansers that are very efficient for removing make-up and grime and leave the skin clean and soft.

· · · ·

Drink a glass of water with a slice of lemon first thing in the morning and drink at least five more large glasses of water (hot or cold) during the day.

· · · ·

Keep coffee and tea to the minimum, no more than 5 cups per day. Any more than two measures of alcohol per day is drying and damaging to the skin. Stop smoking.

· · · ·

Avoid fatty or sugary foods and eat unrefined carbohydrates rather than refined. Try to eat plenty of fresh vegetables and fruit. Eat yogurt regularly.

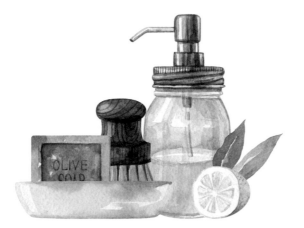

Protect the skin from the elements, wear moisturizer, and wrap up well when going outdoors in the winter, and in the summer always wear a good sunscreen.

. . . .

Remove make-up before going to bed and cleanse the skin thoroughly. Use face masks or exfoliate regularly to remove dead skin cells and freshen the skin.

. . . .

Moisturize the skin after showers or baths, paying attention to the elbows, knees, and heels.

. . . .

Keep the hair clean as dirty hair can be the cause of breakouts on the face and back.

. . . .

Wear natural fabrics next to the skin.

SENSITIVE SKIN

Sensitive skin reacts adversely to external influences. A common cause is cosmetic ingredients, but temperature extremes or poor skin care can also be cited.

. . . .

The symptoms range from dry, flaking skin, rashes, itching, blotches, reddening, and in extreme cases painful swelling.

. . . .

There are two separate problems, irritation and allergy. They show similar skin reactions but have different causes. Irritation is the most frequent problem of sensitive skin. The skin type most prone is usually fair and dry. The cause can be harsh products containing alcohol, strong detergents, or using wrong products for skin type. Sometimes hot water or cold winds can have an irritating effect. The reaction occurs immediately or soon afterwards and worsens if a large amount of the product is applied. The cure is to avoid harsh products. Use baby products or cleansing milk. Never use very hot or cold water, only lukewarm.

. . . .

Allergies occur when the body reacts to a substance that it thinks is harmful. The auto immune system goes into action and sends white blood cells rushing to the skin's surface. This makes the skin red, itchy, and sore. The reaction can take up to a week to appear and sometimes a product can cause an allergy after years of use. Allergies can happen on any skin type.

. . . .

To cure an allergy, first find the cause. A new cosmetic product is an obvious choice; otherwise, all products in use will have to be removed in turn, to find the problem.

. . . .

A food allergy can also cause a skin reaction, so the diet should be checked. Patch tests on the skin with each ingredient can determine which one is causing the reaction.

. . . .

For products used over a long time, but now causing a reaction, it may be worthwhile to contact the manufacturer to ascertain if they have changed the composition of the product.

. . . .

Many teenagers suffer from acne or swollen spots. These result from a bacterial infection causing inflammation around a hair follicle. Although it cannot be prevented, it can be controlled. Avoid squeezing the spots as this can cause scarring to the face.

. . . .

Medical preparations are available from pharmacists and in severe cases special treatment from a doctor will be needed.

. . . .

Avoid changing from one treatment to another if results are not showing in a short time. Most treatments can take up to three months to work and some antibiotic courses can last for six months.

. . . .

Chocolates and fatty food will not make acne worse. It is important to keep the skin clean using a good soap, but extra washing does not help.

. . . .

Do not use steaming if you have bad pustular acne, as heat can spread the problem. Apply a mask daily to clean the skin.

. . . .

For acne, drink 3 cups of freshly brewed nettle tea daily before meals. Pour 1 cup (250 milliliters) of boiling water over 1 heaped tablespoon chopped nettle leaves. Cover and leave for 2 minutes. Strain and sip slowly.

．．．．

All hair follicles on the body have a sebaceous gland and these, triggered by the flow of hormones at puberty, produce sebum or oil to keep the skin and hair in good condition. When these glands produce excess oil the pores become blocked. The trapped sebum results in a blackhead. A deeper blockage produces a whitehead.

．．．．

Keep the skin clean, washing at least 3 times a day. Do not squeeze spots unless you are steam cleansing the face. Then, using a fresh piece of gauze each time, gently squeeze the spots and dab with antiseptic.

．．．．

To loosen blackheads, combine ¼ cup boiling water, 1 teaspoon Epsom salts, and 3 drops iodine, then cool until comfortable to the touch. Soak cotton ball in the mixture and dab on the spots.

．．．．

Remove redness from a spot by mixing 1 teaspoon lemon juice with 1 teaspoon salt, and apply to the spot. Leave for 10 minutes and rinse off.

．．．．

To disguise a spot, dab with calamine lotion before applying foundation or color brown with an eyebrow pencil for an instant beauty mark!

．．．．

To tone down red cheeks or disguise broken veins, wear green tinted moisturizer under foundation.

. . . .

Shaving cream, gel, foam, or soap can irritate the skin and cause redness and/or blotches. Try shaving with your regular conditioner.

FACE SAVERS

Remember that natural ingredients in homemade remedies are as likely to cause reactions as synthetic; always do a patch test on the neck to check that the skin is not sensitive.

. . . .

Face masks either cleanse and revitalize, or nourish and moisturize. Thoroughly cleanse the face as usual. Put a scarf or headband around the head to keep the hair off the face and lotions out of the hair.

. . . .

Face masks or scrubs can leave the face looking very pink for about 30 minutes after removal, so keep this in mind when choosing a time to use one.

. . . .

Masks are more effective if used after a steam cleaning. Lean forward over a bowl of hot water for about three minutes. The steam will relax the skin and open the pores, making it more receptive to the ingredients in the mask. Wipe away any excess moisture and apply the mask. Do not use steam cleaning if you have broken veins on the face.

. . . .

Avoid putting any of the mask preparation on the delicate skin around the eyes. Cover the eyes with pads soaked in iced water while the mask is working.

. . . .

On sensitive skin, if masks are too drying, mix them first with a small quantity of your regular moisturizer.

. . . .

For skin cleansing, apply Milk of Magnesia to the face with cotton balls. Leave on for 10 minutes, remove with a warm face cloth, and apply usual moisturizer.

. . . .

Skin scrubs or exfoliates are available in cream, lotion, or gel form. They contain crushed nuts or oatmeal, which is massaged into the skin, removing the built-up layers of dirt and dead skin cells, leaving the skin soft and smooth.

. . . .

Treat oily and problem skin once or twice a week. On combination skin, only use on the rough or oily areas. Use with caution on sensitive or dry skin.

. . . .

After cleansing the skin thoroughly, use the fingertips to massage the scrub into the skin with a gentle circular movement for two to three minutes. Do not rub too hard as this can irritate the skin or lead to broken veins.

. . . .

Concentrate on the oily areas such as the forehead, sides of the nose, and the chin. Avoid the delicate area around the eyes. Rinse off thoroughly with warm water. Apply a good moisturizer.

BATH TIME

Baths can be used for washing the body, replacing oils, and softening the skin and they can be stimulating or relaxing and relieve tension.

. . . .

Before bathing, use a body scrub to improve circulation, remove dead skin cells, and smooth the skin. Use a loofah or try a scrub of sea salt or oatmeal.

. . . .

An excellent remedy for the skin is to fill a muslin bag with bran or oatmeal and, when taking a bath, soak it in the water by hanging it from the tap. It can be reused a few times.

. . . .

The easiest way to counteract skin dryness is to add oil to the bath. The floating oil clings to the skin and lubricates it. Or rub liquid paraffin all over the body before bathing.

. . . .

For dry itchy skin, add a cup of vinegar to the bath water.

. . . .

"With reasonable care the human body will last a lifetime."
—Arnold Glasgow

To relieve tiredness, add a spoonful of honey to the bath water. For luxury, add a handful of powdered milk or fill a muslin bag with herbs and suspend it in the bath water.

· · · ·

For rough skin on elbows, knees, feet, upper arms, or thighs, pour a handful of coarse salt or granulated sugar and oil onto a damp flannel and rub in brisk circular movements over the troublesome areas.

· · · ·

Washing with soap and water may not always remove the problem of body odor; in these cases, use a deodorant or antiperspirant. A deodorant masks the odor and inhibits bacterial growth to a small extent but does not affect the flow of perspiration. An antiperspirant is composed of chemicals that partially block the pores and reduce the perspiration reaching the skin's surface. Use antiperspirants sparingly, as the body needs to be able to perspire to regulate the body temperature.

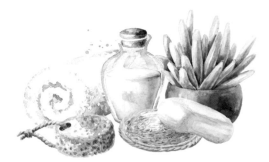

For a natural deodorant, use green leaves, fresh green vegetables (beet tops or spinach), or fresh herbs such as mint. Rub the leaves briskly over the areas that perspire a few times during the day. Or shake 6 drops of lavender oil in 1 pint (600 milliliters) distilled water. Store in a dark-colored bottle in the refrigerator. Apply with cotton balls twice daily where necessary.

PAMPERING YOUR FEET

Feet are not something that most of us think about for much of the time until they become painful, then we think about little else. Most foot problems are caused by badly fitting, or synthetically made footwear and a general lack of foot care.

• • • •

Choose shoes with heels less than 2 inches (5 centimeters) high and try to alternate shoes each day. Shoes should be at least 1 inch (2.5 centimeters) longer than the toes. Very flat shoes as well as too high a heel can cause posture problems, backache, and spinal mismanagement.

• • • •

As people age, the arch of the foot can flatten, pushing the foot forward and outward. This can make it necessary to purchase a larger or broader size of shoe.

• • • •

Shop for shoes in the afternoon to take into account any swelling in the feet during the day.

• • • •

Walk barefoot whenever possible, but try not to expose your feet to cold temperatures.

. . . .

Try not to stand still for long periods, and when playing sports, wear shoes that will properly support the feet.

. . . .

If a lot of time is spent standing or on the feet during the day, occasionally do mini squats by bending the knees a little and straightening the back.

. . . .

To relieve tired feet, take off the shoes during the day, wriggle the toes, and rotate the ankle. Lie down, put the feet up, and massage the legs one at a time from foot to knee.

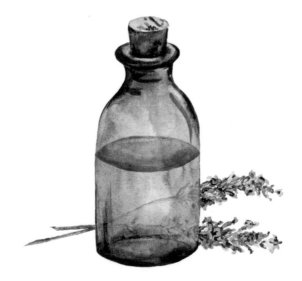

Wash feet daily in warm water but don't soak them for longer than 5 minutes, as the natural oils will tend to dry out. Add a cupful of Epsom salts or bicarbonate of soda with a few drops of lavender, marjoram, tea-tree or rosemary essential oil.

. . . .

A dash of cider vinegar added will help eliminate itching and athlete's foot. Dry well, especially between the toes, and rather than using talcum powder dry off with rubbing alcohol.

. . . .

Give the feet a weekly pedicure. Remove any dead skin from the soles of the feet. Check between the toes for fungal infections and treat if necessary. Use a moisturizing cream on the heels where hard skin is prone to develop.

. . . .

To stimulate circulation, start the day by taking a warm drink of hot water with 1 teaspoon honey and a slice of lemon with fresh ginger root added.

. . . .

For a foot rub, smooth moisturizer or oil onto the soles of the feet and knead them firmly with the thumbs using small circular movements. Then work on the upper part of the feet by pressing and gliding the thumbs between the bones. Squeeze and gently pull each toe. Finish with sweeping upward strokes over each foot.

. . . .

To soften hard skin and revive tired feet, place 2 peppermint tea bags in a bowl of warm water. Soak the feet for 10 minutes, then pat dry with a warm towel. Sprinkle 2 lemon halves with salt and rub over the areas of hard skin. Rinse, and with an old clean blusher brush, paint olive oil over the feet and toes and wrap them in cling film and warm towels. Leave for 10 minutes. Unwrap, and if still oily, pat with tissues.

. . . .

For a foot bath, soak feet in 1 pint (600 milliliters) warm whole milk for 10 minutes, then rinse. Scrub feet with salt-oil mixture of ½ cup coarse salt and ⅓ cup olive oil. Rinse and apply moisturizer and wear thick socks to seal in the softness.

. . . .

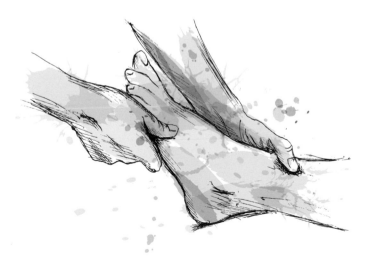

Do not use talcum powder on feet as it can collect around the nails, between the toes, and in any cracks or crevices, causing soreness and infection. Baking soda is a good natural antiperspirant; sprinkle on the feet after washing and drying them.

. . . .

When the skin is soft after washing, check the toenails. Push the cuticles back gently with a fingertip.

. . . .

Toenails should be cut straight across; this helps to strengthen the nails and discourage ingrown toenails.

. . . .

When hard nails are difficult to cut, dab the nail with a cotton ball soaked in peroxide and leave it on for a few minutes.

Feet Complaints

Athlete's foot (tinea pedis) is a yeast-fungal infection and is usually noticed by cracked, red, and itchy skin between the toes. It thrives in warmth and moisture and is exacerbated by sweat or not drying the foot properly after washing. It can spread to the sole of the foot, appearing first as tiny blisters.

. . . .

There are foot and shoe antiperspirant, deodorant sprays, or powders and special shoe insoles obtainable to absorb sweat and clear up infections.

. . . .

For a dormant fungus that frequently breaks out, specific antibiotics can be prescribed by your doctor.

. . . .

To prevent recurrence, wear cotton socks, use a selection of shoes, avoid washing the feet in hot water, and do not walk barefoot at public swimming pools.

. . . .

Verruca is a painful wart that has grown inwards from the pressure of standing. It is caused by a virus. Sometimes a layer of skin grows over the verruca. If it isn't painful then it should be left untouched and it will disappear naturally within two years. It should be covered when attending the public swimming pool. Creams or ointment may be applied and the wart scraped away slowly over a period of weeks. There are courses of herbal tablets available and many of these are very effective. If it is causing discomfort, consult a podiatrist who can remove it surgically by freezing or burning.

. . . .

Sweaty feet are the main cause of smelly feet and this can be mainly due to wearing the wrong footwear. Shoes with synthetic fabric linings do not allow sweat evaporation or absorption, so the foot stays wet. Synthetic socks or stockings have the same effect. Sweaty feet can be more prevalent during puberty due to hormonal changes.

. . . .

To reduce smelly feet, wear loose cotton or wool socks with a close weave to absorb the sweat. If necessary, wear two pairs to increase absorption. Wash socks in the hottest cycle and rinse in well-diluted antiseptic. Chemical-treated socks can also help. If possible, change footwear daily.

. . . .

Wear shoes made from skin or leather, especially the soles. Avoid synthetic linings in shoes and avoid wearing trainers for long periods. When weather conditions permit, wear sandals or go barefoot.

. . . .

For smelly, sweaty feet, apply zinc and castor oil cream nightly for a week. Reuse when required. Or brew two tea bags in 1 pint (600 milliliters) water for 15 minutes. Pour the tea into a bowl containing 2 pints (1.2 liters) cool water. Soak the feet for 5 minutes daily until the problem diminishes. Then soak them periodically. This can also help ease chilblains.

. . . .

To ease puffy feet, lie flat on the floor with the feet raised above head level on a cushion for 30 minutes.

. . . .

Calluses are mainly found on the ball and heel of the foot. They are areas of hard thick skin caused by badly fitted shoes. To prevent calluses, moisturize the feet frequently.

. . . .

Dead skin can be removed by pumice stone or special skin remover cream; use with care so that the skin is not broken.

. . . .

Corns are hard lumps of thick dead skin. They are generally found on the top or the side of the toes where they rub against the shoes. If they hurt, soak the foot in warm soapy water for 10 minutes. Rub the corn with an emery board twice a week after soaking.

. . . .

Special corn adhesive bandages are available that will prevent the shoe irritating the corn. Never cut a corn with a razor blade as you may get it infected. Instead, if very troublesome, go to a podiatrist and let them trim it with sterilized instruments.

. . . .

To get rid of corn and calluses, make a vinegar compress by soaking a piece of stale bread in cider vinegar, and tape over the problem area overnight.

. . . .

Chilblains are shiny red swellings on the toes. They are caused by poor circulation as a result of standing outdoors in the cold. When feet warm up they become painful and itchy. Caffeine, alcohol, and nicotine are vasoconstrictors and will make them worse.

. . . .

Rub chilblains with a slice of onion dipped in salt. Avoid scratching or the skin will break and become infected.

. . . .

Calamine lotion will also help soothe the irritation. Or add 1 tablespoon dried mustard to a bowl of hot water. Soak the feet for 10 minutes.

. . . .

To prevent chilblains, wear warm socks and well-insulated shoes. Keep the legs warm as well to increase blood circulation. Do not warm the feet directly from the fire or on a hot water bottle. Exercise the legs and feet.

. . . .

Hammer-toe is caused by a shortening of the tendons that control toe movements. It usually affects the second or third toe. The toe is bent downwards and the toe knuckle is usually enlarged, drawing the toe back. Over time, the joint enlarges and stiffens as it rubs against shoes. Your balance may be affected.

. . . .

Wear properly fitted, roomy footwear. A podiatrist can provide padding for the toes and, if the damage is very severe, surgery may be necessary.

. . . .

Ingrown toenails dig into the flesh at either side of the toe and can be very painful. The big toe is the one usually affected. Sometimes the surrounding area of skin is red and swollen and maybe even cut by the nail.

. . . .

If the area is infected, then consult a doctor. Otherwise soak the foot in warm water for 10 minutes. Lift the ingrown part of the nail with a nail file and slip a piece of cotton wool under it. Remove and replace with fresh cotton wool daily until the nail grows beyond the corner of the toe.

. . . .

Before going to bed, either put a small wedge of lemon on the toenail or take the skin/membrane from eggshells and wrap, wet side down around the toe, securing with an adhesive bandage and a sock. In the morning, the nail should be soft enough to ease it away from the skin so that you can trim it. Always cut the nail straight across and not any shorter than the toe; do not round off the corners. Avoid narrow shoes.

. . . .

Bunions are growths over the bone at the first joint of the big toes. Since there is a dislocation of the joint, the big toe may be tight against the second toe or even overlapping it. Tight, narrow shoes aggravate bunions and they can be very painful.

. . . .

Avoid wearing high-heeled narrow shoes and, whenever possible, go barefoot. Pads to separate the toes and reduce the pressure can be purchased at drug stores. In severe cases, surgery involving the reconstruction of the toe joint will probably be recommended by your doctor or podiatrist. Bunions tend to be hereditary.

. . . .

Spurs are calcium growths that develop on the bones of the feet. They are caused by muscle strain in the feet. Standing for long periods of time, wearing badly fitting shoes, or being overweight can make spurs worse. They can be very painful or painless. Treatments include using foot supports, heel pads, and heel cups. Sometimes surgery is required.

. . . .

Painful balls of the feet can be caused by high heels as they throw the weight forward, putting pressure on the balls of the feet or metatarsus, causing pain. Other causes can be high arches, or prominent metatarsal bones.

. . . .

To ease the pain, apply an ice pack or bathe the feet in cold running water. Wear shoes with lower heels, and check with a pharmacist or podiatrist for special insoles or pads that will help relieve the pressure. Sometimes calf-stretching exercises help.

. . . . .

Fallen arches, or flat foot, is a condition of the foot when the entire sole rests on the ground when the person is standing. Sometimes no discomfort accompanies flat foot, but fallen arches may cause misalignment of other foot structures resulting in aching feet and sometimes back pain, and the discomfort can be increased by prolonged standing.

. . . . .

Flat foot may be inherited or may be caused by rickets, obesity, metabolic disorder, debilitating disease, or faulty footwear. A podiatrist can fit an arch support in the shoe and prescribe strengthening exercises. In severe cases, surgery may be used to correct the problem.

. . . . .

Pain at the back of the heel is usually caused by changing from high heels to flats or bare feet. The cord-like Achilles tendon at the back of the heel can become over-stretched and result in tendonitis. The pain can run up the leg to the back of the knee. For relief, apply an ice pack for 10 minutes.

. . . . .

To avoid further damage, do calf-stretching exercises for two minutes every day for two weeks; standing barefooted, place the palms of the hands against the wall and stand arm's length back from it. Keeping the back straight and feet flat on the floor, bend the arms until the nose touches the wall. Push back slowly and repeat.

. . . . .

After prolonged barefoot walking, the feet may suffer from a painful area or aching. Examine carefully for an embedded thorn or sliver of broken glass that has become infected. Prolonged vigorous walking can cause minute hairline fractures in small foot bones. Rest and bathe to aid healing.

. . . .

For foot blisters, squeeze a little white liquid of a dandelion onto the blister and then cover it with a bandage. Only use dandelions that have not been sprayed with pesticides and if this liquid causes any discomfort, wash it off immediately. You could have a skin sensitivity to the substance.

Hard-working Hands

No matter how much outward care is lavished on the hands, if the body is not properly nourished, the fingernails will be the first indicator of poor diet. Drinking 8 glasses of water daily keeps the body properly hydrated and prevents dry skin and flaky nails.

When using any implements on infected nails, it is important to keep them away from healthy nails.

. . . .

Buff nails with a chamois leather buffer to stimulate circulation and strengthen them.

. . . .

Straight acetone used to remove nail varnish can dry and split nails. Nail enamel removers have special oils added to prevent damage to the nails. Refrain from peeling off old enamel as a layer of nail can also come off.

. . . .

"Beautiful hands are those that do deeds that are noble, good, and true."
—Unknown

To avoid nails breaking, keep them fairly short, especially when using a keyboard. Use a pencil to dial numbers on the telephone and never use nails to pry open compacts, or to untie laces or string.

. . . . .

Shape nails by filing into smooth, rounded ovals, but leave growth at the sides so that the nails don't in-grow and cause infection. File one way only, from side to center. Back and forth filing shreds nail fibers.

. . . . .

Do not bite the nails as this leaves them ragged and unsightly; deterrent solutions are available to stop the habit.

. . . . .

Leave nails free of nail varnish occasionally. Constant use, especially without a colorless base-coat, can cause yellowing of the nails. Refrain from smoking, as this will also stain the nails. Stained nails should be brushed twice daily with lemon juice followed by white wine vinegar, then massage with almond oil.

. . . . .

An excellent conditioner for nails is a soak for 10 minutes in hot almond, castor, wheat-germ, or baby oil.

. . . . .

To help nails strengthen and grow, mix 1 tablespoon almond oil with a packet of unflavored gelatin, or blend 1 tablespoon cider vinegar with 1 tablespoon olive oil and 1 egg yolk. Store in an airtight container at room temperature. Massage into the nails twice daily to restore brittle nails.

. . . .

For a moisturizing nail cream, mix together 1 teaspoon each of avocado, liquid honey, and 1 egg yolk. Rub into and around the fingernails, then rinse off after 30 minutes.

. . . .

Massaging or buffing nails helps improve circulation and stimulates growth.

. . . .

Buff nails with a little almond oil or beeswax on a piece of soft, closely woven, natural cloth wrapped around a cotton ball or with a nail buffer which has a soft pad covered in fine leather.

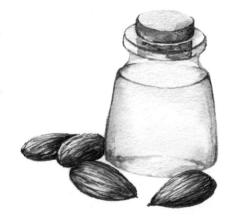

Never use cuticle scissors; they can easily nip the skin and cause an infection.

. . . . .

Gently push back the cuticles with the towel when washing the hands. Or use a popsicle stick wrapped in cotton wool. Rub cuticles with hand cream or special cuticle cream.

. . . . .

To make cuticle cream, mix 2 tablespoons each of pineapple juice and egg yolk with ½ teaspoon cider vinegar, soak the nails for 30 minutes, rinse off. Use nightly to "feed" the growing nails.

. . . . .

To fix a broken nail, use a teabag, nail glue, and some cotton wool. Soak a small tuft of cotton wool in glue and pull it across the split. Place a small piece of teabag (minus the tea) on the glued area, allow to dry, then buff up as usual.

. . . . .

White flecks or "chalk marks" on the nails are just immature cells which didn't become transparent. It has nothing to do with lack of calcium. They can be more prevalent after injury to a nail or after manicuring. If the finger just below the nail was knocked, a white spot can appear on the nail up to six months later.

. . . . .

Brittle or chipped nails are not caused by lack of calcium either. They can be caused by anemia or circulatory problems, but the more common cause is from household cleaners and detergents, so wear rubber gloves when washing.

. . . . .

Nails that are dark pink at the top and pale at the bottom may mean there is a kidney problem. Kidney problems cause water retention and this makes the nail bed swell, cutting off the blood supply to the base of the nail.

. . . .

If pale nails are not hereditary this can also be a sign of kidney problems that cause anemia or lack of iron. Pale nails could also mean a lack of protein in the diet.

. . . .

Blue nails can be a sign of poor circulation that may be due to a heart disorder, high blood pressure, arteriosclerosis, varicose veins, or a blood vessel disorder.

. . . .

Spoon nails may be a sign of anemia since lack of iron in the diet can leave the nails flaky and easily bent. A small indentation can be caused by the nail growth being interrupted by a knock or infection.

. . . .

Clubbed nails—when the tips are bulbous—can indicate lung disease, cirrhosis of the liver, or inflammatory bowel disease.

. . . .

Yellow, thickening nails, are usually a sign of ageing but can also be a symptom of psoriasis, or a sign of lung, thyroid, or lymphatic problems.

. . . .

It takes five months for a complete nail to grow and they grow more quickly during the summer months. They also grow more quickly on the hand you use most and on the longer fingers.

• • • •

For hygienic reasons, hands should be kept clean and as germ-free as possible.

• • • •

When washing hands, remove all rings, use lukewarm water and a little soap, rinse well, and dry thoroughly, especially between the fingers.

• • • •

Apply a barrier cream to hands before commencing chores or immersing them in water containing detergents.

• • • •

Wear plastic or rubber gloves when using strong detergents, chemical products, or when working with spirits, turpentine, dry-cleaning fluid, or petrol.

• • • •

An exfoliating scrub and using a good hand cream afterwards will keep the skin on the hands soft and remove any hyper-pigmentation or age spots.

• • • •

Banish age spots by mixing 1 teaspoon boric acid with a little lemon juice. Cover the age spot with the mixture and cover with an adhesive bandage. Leave for a few minutes then wash off with lemon juice. Apply a few times until the spot disappears.

. . . .

Or mix together 2 tablespoons fine oatmeal, 1 tablespoon full-fat plain yogurt, 2 teaspoons almond oil, and 2 teaspoons lime juice. Stir to a paste and spread over the back of the hands. Leave for 10 minutes and rub in some hand cream. Use three times a week.

. . . .

For a hand cleanser, add equal amounts of lemon juice and olive oil to 1 tablespoon caster sugar until it is moistened. Rub the mixture into the hands and around the nails for a few minutes. Rinse off with tepid water. This mixture will remove many stains; it also softens and whitens the hands.

. . . .

Stains on hands can be removed by rubbing them with the inside skin of a lemon or orange; also try a slice of potato.

. . . .

Rich hand creams will be more effective if used at night and the hands covered with a pair of cotton gloves. Lighter cream should be applied frequently during the day. When applying hand creams, always massage the hands well.

. . . .

Dry cracked hands can be soothed with a mixture of grated potato and olive oil. Apply to the skin, leave for 10 minutes, and rinse off.

. . . .

Warm two soft washcloths in the microwave. Rub moisturizing cream or the oil from a vitamin E capsule into the hands. Wrap the hands in the hot washcloths and relax for 10 minutes.

. . . .

Soften rough hands or feet by rubbing first with a pumice stone, then soak in warm water with 2 teaspoons Epsom salts added, for 5 minutes. Then rub with warm olive oil. Do not use a pumice stone on wet skin as it can slough off more skin than is comfortable.

. . . .

Cover a small cupful of bran flakes with 1 pint (600 milliliters) boiling water. Cover and allow to cool for 10 hours. Strain and add 4 tablespoons cider vinegar. Stir well, bottle, and label. Rub well into chapped hands until they feel dry.

. . . .

Mix equal amounts of pure lemon juice, glycerin, and rosewater and store in an airtight glass bottle. Massage generously into the hands and wrists. Or warm enough almond oil to soak dry, chapped hands in for 15 minutes.

. . . .

Warm 1½ teaspoons clear honey until runny. Remove from the heat and blend in ½ teaspoon cider vinegar, 8 tablespoons rosewater, and 4 tablespoons glycerin. Bottle, label, and use regularly on chapped hands.

. . . .

For a rich moisturizer, in a double saucepan melt and blend together 4 tablespoons coconut oil, 6 tablespoons sweet almond oil, and 6 tablespoons shredded beeswax. Add 6 tablespoons glycerin and stir slowly until the mixture looks smooth. Pot and label.

To make a moisturizer for hands, combine to a smooth paste 1 tablespoon honey, 2 tablespoons ground almonds, and 1 egg yolk. Apply to the hands and leave on for 10 minutes. Rinse off and dry well. Apply hand cream.

. . . .

Give hands a daily workout:
- Rub the palms of the hands together until they are warm.
- Make a tight fist with each hand and then slowly stretch out all the fingers as far as possible. Repeat 5–6 times.
- With the fingers extended, rotate the hands, first clockwise, then anti-clockwise 5–6 times.
- Play the scales on an imaginary piano for 30 seconds.
- With the palms of the hands pressed together, gently open and close the fingers as far as possible. Place two large sheets of newspaper on a flat surface and, using one hand at a time, screw up the paper until it is a tight ball. This improves the grip.
- To relax the hands after the exercise, let the hands hang loose and shake them gently from the wrist.

. . . .

Warts are a contagious growth on the top layer of the skin and usually affect areas of skin prone to injury such as hands, elbows, face, knees, and scalp. They can be round, flat-topped, or finger-like projections and tend to disappear spontaneously within a year. Regression of warts can be aided with wart-dissolving liquids, freezing, or heat treatment.

. . . .

To help get rid of warts use one of the following:

- Chop a piece of onion and cover with salt. Leave overnight and dab the wart twice daily with the resulting juice.
- Apply 2 drops tea tree oil morning and night to kill the virus.
- Cover the wart overnight with a small piece of banana skin; tape the furry side down over the wart.
- Apply vitamin E–enriched oil and cover with an adhesive bandage. Repeat 3 times daily. This can take several weeks to work.
- Put some crushed garlic onto the wart and cover with an adhesive bandage; after a day the wart should blister and fall off.
- Pick a dandelion and dab the sap onto the wart; the best sap is found just underneath the head of the flower. The wart immediately turns black and, if continued once a day for 9 days, the wart disappears, leaving clear soft skin.

SUNBATHING

People with pale complexions should avoid the mid-day sun.

. . . .

Remember sand and concrete surfaces can reflect the sun back at you causing the skin to burn more easily.

. . . .

Use waterproof sunscreen when swimming, as the body will still catch the sun. Reapply hourly to maintain protection.

. . . .

It can take up to four hours for sunburn to show on the skin, so don't be fooled by the pale skin color. Use a stronger sun protection factor on the face, shoulders, ankles, and feet as these areas are easily burned.

. . . .

A haze over the sun does not prevent the ultraviolet rays from coming through and causing burning.

. . . .

Most sunscreen products have a sun protection factor rating. Generally, people with pale blue or green eyes need a strong factor while those with hazel or brown eyes need less.

. . . .

The sun dries out the skin, so it's important to moisturize after sunbathing. After-sun products help to lock in moisture and reduce the skin peeling.

. . . .

If you get sunburned, the skin will be red and feel tight and sore. Soothe the skin with calamine lotion, cider vinegar, or aloe.

. . . .

Drink plenty of liquid if you feel dizzy or have nausea.

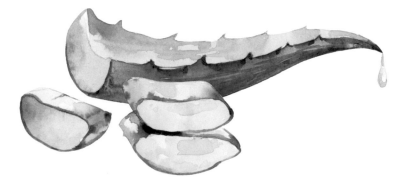

Increase vitamin C intake. It makes your skin less sensitive to the sun. Foods rich in vitamin C include citrus fruits, apples, green onions, black and red currant, rosehip tea.

. . . .

Tanning bed treatment before sunbathing does not stop the sun burning. Like the sun itself, tanning beds will accelerate skin ageing and increase the chance of skin cancer.

TUMMY TROUBLES

Effective chewing is important for digestion as it increases the saliva flow in the mouth. Only put small amounts of food into the mouth. Eat slowly and taste the food. Chew with the mouth closed.

. . . .

Saliva has many functions:
- It is important to the sense of taste.
- It lubricates the food so that it can be swallowed easily.
- It rinses the mouth of any food left after swallowing.
- It neutralizes acids.
- It produces the enzyme ptyalin that starts the breakdown of starch to sugar.

. . . .

Learn to relax when eating. Put the knife and fork down between mouthfuls. A glass of wine with a meal is relaxing and will aid digestion. Anxious or sensitive people are more susceptible to indigestion. Stress causes the stomach to produce high quantities of acid.

. . . .

"The good thing about swallowing pride is that it doesn't choke you."
—Unknown

Have a short rest after a meal to give the digestive system more energy to work on the food you've eaten. Have regular, daily exercise—even a short walk.

. . . .

Take small meals at regular intervals. The stomach is constantly producing acid. Irregular meals means the acid has long periods with no food to digest and this causes a burning sensation in the stomach: indigestion.

. . . .

Avoid foods you know cause you to have indigestion.

. . . .

If prone to indigestion, avoid smoking, alcohol, aspirin, strong coffee, and tea as they can cause irritation to the stomach lining.

. . . .

Avoid overeating, and supper should be several hours before bedtime. For nighttime indigestion, raise the head-end of the bed about 4 inches (10 centimeters).

. . . .

Antacid medicine or sips of soda water will help relieve symptoms, or sip a glass of warm water with 1 tablespoon honey and 1 tablespoon cider vinegar added. If constantly bothered with indigestion or worried about frequent stomach pains it is advisable to visit the doctor.

. . . .

For constipation, take syrup of figs. Simmer 8 chopped figs in ½ pint (300 milliliters) water until soft. Stir 2 ounces (50 grams) brown sugar and a pinch ginger. Blend and keep in the refrigerator. Take 1–2 tablespoons daily.

GOING THROUGH THE MOTIONS

The digestive system is the key to good health and impacts the physical and mental wellbeing of the body.

. . . .

Frequency of passing stools varies from once or twice a day to three times a week. If there is a change in bowel habits you should seek medical attention.

. . . .

To determine transit time from consumption of food to expulsion, eat either beets or sweet corn and note when traces are seen in the stool. A hundred hours is slow while 10 hours is fast. The normal is anything in between these times.

. . . .

Stools are a very good indicator of what is happening inside our body, so if they are hard and difficult to pass, this means your calorie intake is too low and you are not getting enough essential fats. You need to drink more fluids, take a spoonful of olive oil before bedtime, and improve the diet.

. . . .

Runny or mushy stools shows a high alcohol intake or you are stressed. Eat yogurt and high-fiber food. Learn to relax.

. . . .

Lumpy stools indicate poor digestion, resulting in certain nutrients not being absorbed. Relax before meals and eat slowly.

. . . .

Very dark stools means the stool has spent too long in transit. Eat more fruit and vegetables.

. . . .

Pale stools show that an excessively fatty meal was consumed, probably with alcohol. If pale stools are associated with dark urine, this could indicate liver disease. Drink plenty of herbal tea, and eat small meals of whole grains and protein. Seek medical attention if pale stools persist.

. . . .

Stools covered in excess mucus can indicate you may have an inflammatory bowel problem. This can be due to consuming high levels of processed food. Seek medical attention and improve the diet.

. . . .

Difficult to flush means the fat content of the stool is high. Too much food, high in saturated fat, has been consumed. It can also be a symptom of pancreatic disease. Reduce the intake of fatty and processed food. Eat more fresh vegetables. Seek medical attention if the problem persists.

. . . .

When bothered with diarrhea, grate a peeled apple onto a plate
and leave for 20 minutes until the apple turns brown, then eat it.
Or drink a cup of unsweetened black tea.

TREASURE CHEST

Never buy a bra without trying it on first. A badly fitting bra can
contribute to health problems. When a bra is too big, the breasts
can droop and encourage poor posture, resulting in neck pain,
backache, headache, and tingling in the arms.

. . . .

When the under-band is too tight there will be pressure marks
under the cups. If the cup size is too small the extreme pressure
across the cup can damage the breast tissue.

. . . .

To get the correct fit, lean forward when trying on a bra and make
sure all the breast tissue fits into the cup. Then lift up the straps
when still in this position.

. . . .

Ensure the bra is fitted on the middle hook so there's a bit of give
if it shrinks in the wash or stretches with wear.

. . . .

Lycra-mix fabric bras are best for keeping their shape. Different
bra styles fit better than others.

. . . .

Do not wear an under-wired bra when pregnant as it has the
potential to stop milk flow.

. . . .

"The happiest people don't always have the best of everything, they just make the best of everything."
—Unknown

For small breasts, choose light support, and for medium breasts choose a bra with under-wiring or side support. Large breasts need bras with deep side bands slightly padded and with wide straps for good support.

. . . .

To measure your bra size, first measure under the bust. If the number is even, add 4 inches. If it is odd, add 5 inches. A measurement of 30 inches gives a bra size of 34". Pendulous breasts should be measured with a bra on.

. . . .

For cup size, measure the fullest part of the bust. The difference in inches between the fullest part of the bust and under-bust measurements gives the cup size.

. . . .

When bra and cup size measure the same the cup size is A.
If there is:
- 1" difference the cup size is B
- 2" difference the cup size is C
- 3" difference the cup size is D
- 4" difference the cup size is DD
- 5" difference the cup size is E
- 6" difference the cup size is F

. . . .

Check that the cup completely covers the breast. Bulges at the top or sides indicate the cup is too small. Neither should the sides of the cup wrinkle because the breast does not fill it.

. . . .

The back of the bra should stay down on the body. If it slips up then the bra size may be too large, it may be hooked too loosely, or the straps may be adjusted too tightly.

. . . .

The bra should be snug but not tight around the body. If it cuts into the skin, the back size is too small or the back closure needs to be loosened. The garment is too tight if you cannot slip your finger easily behind the bra strap.

. . . .

The center of the bra should lie flat against the breast-bone. If it stretches away from the body, the cup size is too small.

. . . .

Straps should be adjusted to support the breasts comfortably without pressure. Check the width of the strap for your personal preference.

. . . .

Always wear a bra when exercising or playing sports. Most sports bras are made from soft cotton and are seamless across the nipples to prevent friction. Some sports bras have no cups and are like short vests that bind the breasts close to the chest.

. . . .

The only way to achieve a smaller bust is to do aerobic exercises which burn fatty tissue from all over the body. Breasts are composed of a great deal of fatty tissue. Disregard creams or miracle cures, as they don't work.

. . . .

Exercising the pectorals (chest), seratus (under the bust), deltoids (shoulders), latissimus dorsi (back), triceps, and biceps (upper arms) will make the breasts appear firmer and improve posture, lifting the breasts up and out.

. . . .

Splash breasts daily with ice-cold water to tone and firm.

. . . .

To tone the breasts, mix together 1 tablespoon aloe vera gel, 5 drops juniper essential oil, and 4 drops each of lemon essential oil and geranium oil. Bottle, label, and keep in the refrigerator. Apply to the breasts daily. Do not use while breastfeeding.

. . . .

To firm breasts and tighten the skin, mix 1 teaspoon vitamin E oil with 1 tablespoon yogurt and an egg. Massage this mixture into breasts and wear an old bra over the mixture for at least twenty minutes. Rinse off with warm water.

. . . .

Breasts should be massaged at least once a month to promote blood flow and stimulate the lymphatic system. Break open a vitamin E capsule and gently massage into the skin. Or use chamomile or geranium essential oil diluted with wheat germ or almond oil.

. . . .

Cabbage leaves help to relieve the pain of mastitis in the breasts. Remove the central stalk of the large outside leaves. Bruise the leaves with a rolling pin and warm in a steamer or microwave before applying to the affected breast or line a bra with them. Drink at least ½ pint (300 milliliters) soy milk a day.

. . . .

Breasts should be checked regularly. Since many women have lumpy breasts, particularly before a period, checks should be made at the end of the period.

. . . .

To do your own breast check: Stand in front of a mirror and look carefully at your breasts. Look for any unusual increase in the size, dimpling, or changes in the skin texture, changes in the nipples or discharges from them, and also take notice of any unusual protruding veins. Put the hands behind the head and swivel from side to side, to view the breasts from different angles. Lower and raise the arms to check your breasts move together. Lean forward and examine each breast for any changes in outline or puckering. Lie down and get into a comfortable position. Start with the left breast and using the flat of the fingers, not the tips, press gently on the breast working in circular movements from the outside of the breast in towards the nipple. Feel for changes in the breasts; some growths feel like peas and can move a little when pressed. Others are more fixed or are like a sort of thickness. Finally, check for any lumps along the top of the collarbone and in the armpit. If any changes are noticed in the breasts, unusual swelling of the upper arm, or enlarged glands in the armpit, seek medical attention immediately.

. . . .

If a thin bra strap is too tight and digs into the shoulder, it puts downward pressure on the cervical nerve that runs from the neck to the shoulder. Damage to this nerve can cause frequent headaches, neck pain, or numbness. Over time, pain can radiate from the shoulder, down the arms, and into the hands. Tight bra straps are especially hazardous for full-busted women, but all women are susceptible.

Natural Beauty Treatments

NATURAL BEAUTY TREATMENTS

For years, natural things like petals, herbs, leaves, roots, fruit, and vegetables have been used to make beauty preparations.

. . . .

With homemade beauty treatments, always do a patch test in case of an allergic reaction to the ingredients.

. . . .

Use stainless steel or enamel containers to prepare treatments. Avoid non-stick or aluminum as these may alter the nature of the ingredients.

. . . .

Sterilize the jars or bottles you use to store the preparation. If the potion gets infected with bacteria it will go off quickly and could harm the skin.

. . . .

Date and label the jars. Glass jars and bottles are the best containers as metal may taint the potion. The lids should preferably be screw-top and airtight.

. . . .

Homemade mixtures contain no preservatives or stabilizers, so only make up small quantities and store in the refrigerator. Unless otherwise stated, throw away all preparations after four days.

. . . .

"In nature, nothing is perfect and everything is perfect. Trees can be contorted, bent in weird ways, and they're still beautiful."
—Alice Walker

Always use fresh ingredients and measure them carefully, as accuracy will produce more successful results. If the ingredients are not available growing wild or in your garden, you will find them in your local supermarket, greengrocer, health food shop, or chemist.

· · · ·

Roots, herbs, and leaves can be used in two different ways. An infusion is made by pouring 1 pint (600 milliliters) of boiling water over 1 ounce (25 grams) of the essential ingredient. Leave to infuse for at least 30 minutes, cool, and strain. Decoction is extraction by boiling and is used for roots and seeds. Boil 1 ounce (25 grams) of the ingredient in 1.75 pint (1 liter) water. Simmer until the water is reduced by half, cool, and strain.

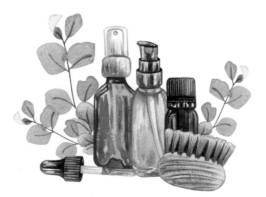

Extracts that can be made are:

- Cinnamon for stimulating the appetite.
- Cloves for soothing toothache.
- Dandelion for brightening dull skin.
- Garlic relieves congestion and improves digestion.
- Marigold helps clear skin and is beneficial on oily skin.
- Mint aids fresh breath.
- Parsley helps dandruff and will darken hair.
- Rhubarb root can highlight mousy hair.
- Rosemary is refreshing for the feet.
- Sage is useful to close open pores.
- Thyme will make an invigorating scalp shampoo.

USING HERBS AND PLANTS

Grow your own herbs; window boxes can hold a good variety. Use them for cooking as well as beauty or health treatments.

• • • •

For an herbal bath, heat 1 pint (600 milliliters) cider vinegar and 1 pint (600 milliliters) water, but do not boil. Add 6 tablespoons (90 milliliters) chopped mixed herbs (elderflower, eucalyptus, lemon balm, mint) and simmer for 10 minutes. Strain and add to the bath water.

• • • •

To soothe under-eye puffiness, boil a handful of chopped rosehips in ½ pint (300 milliliters) water for 10 minutes. Cool until just warm. Soak two pads of cotton wool in the solution and cover the eyes with these for 15 minutes.

• • • •

Facial steam baths can open up your pores and increase circulation. Do not use this treatment if you have sensitive skin or thread veins on your face. Pour 1 pint (600 milliliters) of boiling water over a handful of any mixed dried herbs in a large bowl. Keep covered while cleansing the face thoroughly. Drape a towel loosely over the head and, holding the face at least nine inches above the water, steam for 5–10 minutes. Pat dry and wipe over with a soothing lotion.

. . . .

Natural parsley juice (or parsley infusion) mixed with an equal amount of lemon juice, orange juice, and red currant juice and applied under your favorite cream will help keep freckles invisible.

. . . .

For blackheads, soak a sprig of parsley in a cup of mineral water for 12 hours. Apply the strained lotion on the affected areas with cotton wool.

. . . .

Parsley face pack: Boil a handful of fresh parsley in ½ pint (300 milliliters) water for 10 minutes. Strain and cool, then mix with 1 tablespoon honey and a stiffly beaten egg white. Smooth onto the face and leave for 15–20 minutes. Wash off with warm water.

. . . .

Mud face pack: Pour 1 cup (250 milliliters) of boiling water over 2 tablespoons dried sage and parsley. Leave for 10 minutes and strain. Mix 1 tablespoon of the infusion with 1 whisked egg white. Add enough Fuller's Earth or kaolin to make a paste for a face mask; use the remaining liquid as an antiseptic toner.

. . . .

Collect blackberry leaves from an area free from weed killer or other sprays. Make an infusion with a handful of crushed leaves in ½ pint (300 milliliter) boiling water. Leave for an hour and strain. For several nights, use all of the infusion each night in the bath, to revitalize tired, dry skin. You can follow the same steps with raspberry leaves. To darken grey hair, use the infusion as a final rinse and let it run into a bowl so that it can be used repeatedly.

. . . .

Blackberry leaf tea is also very beneficial; sweeten heated infusion with sugar to taste.

. . . .

As a skin cleanser, mix ¼ pint (150 milliliters) of the infusion with ¼ pint (150 milliliters) of plain yogurt and apply as usual. The remaining infusion can be used as a skin toner.

. . . .

Lotion for greasy skin: Make an infusion of either lavender, lemon balm, rosemary, or yarrow. Mix ¼ pint (150 milliliters) of the cool, strained infusion with ¼ pint (150 milliliters) plain yogurt.

. . . .

Lotion for dry skin: Soak 3 tablespoons chamomile, elderflower, or meadowsweet in ½ pint (300 milliliter) fresh milk for an hour. Heat gently to almost boiling, cool, strain, bottle, cap, and store in the refrigerator.

. . . .

*"Beauty is an experience, nothing else.
It is not a fixed pattern or an arrangement of features.
It is something felt, a glow or a communicated sense of fineness. What ails
us is that our sense of beauty
is so bruised and blunted, we miss all the best."
—D. H. Lawrence*

Toner for greasy skin: Pour ¼ pint (150 milliliters) of boiling water over 2 tablespoons chopped sage, and allow to cool. Strain into ¼ pint (150 milliliters) cider vinegar.

. . . .

Toner for dry skin: Soak 2 tablespoons dried elderflower, marigold, marshmallow, or meadowsweet in 1 pint (600 milliliters) boiling water. Cover and leave to cool for one hour, then strain, bottle, and cap.

. . . .

For a foot bath, add a handful each of dried thyme and peppermint leaves to 1 pint (600 milliliters) water. Bring to a boil and simmer for 5 minutes. Add enough cold water to cool to a comfortable temperature. Soak the feet in this preparation for 10–15 minutes.

. . . .

Alternatively, pour 1 pint (500 milliliters) boiling water over 2 tablespoons fresh nettle leaves and flowers. Leave to infuse for 2–3 hours. The longer the infusion, the stronger the solution. Use the solution warm and soak the feet for at least five minutes.

Using Oils & Honey

Essential oils are extracted from wild or cultivated plants. Many of these oils are expensive due to the complicated extraction process. Purchase essential oils from a reputable outlet. Check the label to know the percentage of pure essence the oil contains.

. . . .

The majority of essential oils should be diluted with a base oil. Generally only a few drops are required. Use good quality base oils such as cold-pressed sweet almond, sunflower, corn, olive, jojoba, wheat germ, or grapeseed oil.

. . . .

Essential oils should keep their potency for 1–2 years, but once diluted in a base oil they will only last for 3 months.

. . . .

Store at a fairly constant room temperature in corked dark glass bottles. Adding some vitamin E or wheat germ oil to the mixture can prolong potency.

. . . .

To use essential oils in the bath, make sure the bathroom is warm and the doors and windows closed. Dilute 4–6 drops of essential oil in 2 tablespoons base oil or milk and add to the bath. Soak the body for 10 minutes, breathing deeply to inhale the vapors.

. . . .

Massage is a very effective method for the oil to be absorbed into the body. Dilute 4–6 drops of essential oil with 2 teaspoons almond or grapeseed oil to avoid causing irritation to the skin. Massage the body for at least 10 minutes.

. . . .

Inhaling steam that is infused with certain essential oils, such as eucalyptus, can be beneficial to respiratory health. Add a few drops to a bowl of hot water. Put a towel over your head and lean over the bowl about 9 inches (22 centimeters) above the water. Breathe deeply to inhale the vapors. This procedure is not advisable for people with sensitive skin.

. . . .

To gargle, add 2–3 drops of tea-tree, lavender, or chamomile to 1 teaspoon vodka and dilute with 2 tablespoons water. Swish around the mouth and throat then spit out.

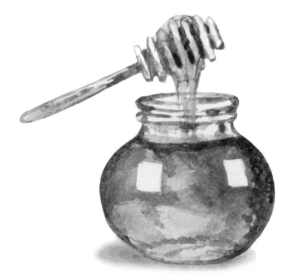

Basil essential oil is an uplifting oil that helps to relieve tension and stress. It can also aid indigestion and flatulence if you dilute with a base oil and massage the tummy area. It will alleviate respiratory infections and has insect repellent qualities. Avoid basil oil during pregnancy.

• • • •

Bergamot relieves tension and irritability. It is also an antiseptic, so it can be used to treat sore throats, mouth ulcers, and bad breath when used as a gargle.

• • • •

Cedarwood is an uplifting and soothing oil. It is an astringent, so it's good for oily skin, greasy hair, acne, dandruff, and scalp irritations. It can also help to relieve cystitis.

• • • •

Chamomile is useful for the treatment of many skin complaints and promotes the healing of burns, cuts, and inflammation. It is effective for the relief of period pains, headaches, insomnia, toothache, and anxiety.

• • • •

Clove is a powerful antiseptic and mild analgesic, excellent for treating gum infections and toothaches. Also valuable for respiratory problems such as bronchitis and skin conditions like scabies or athlete's foot.

• • • •

Eucalyptus has great disinfectant, antiseptic, stimulant, and healing properties. As a natural decongestant, it is a good aid for respiratory complaints. Its analgesic properties can be used for insect bites, ringworm, shingles, or muscular aches.

. . . .

Lavender is beneficial in the treatment of minor burns and scalds, wounds, varicose ulcers, or any healing problem. It can be used for the treatment of muscular aches and pains, digestive problems, genito-urinary problems, and it can have a soothing effect for headaches and pre-menstrual tension. It is one of the oils that can be applied undiluted to the skin.

. . . .

Lemongrass will help revive a sluggish digestive system, relieve muscular aches, and is useful to treat thrush and athlete's foot. Will deter mosquitoes when it is applied to the skin, diluted in a base oil.

. . . .

Rose increases vitality and is useful for menopausal symptoms. Excellent for older skin to soothe away dryness.

. . . .

Rosemary is excellent for stimulating the circulation and useful in the treatment of muscular sprains and aches. It is good for the treatment of skin and hair problems, especially dandruff. This oil is also known to improve concentration and memory problems.

. . . .

Tea Tree is antiseptic, disinfectant, anti-bacterial, anti-fungal, and anti-viral. With all these qualities it can be used to treat respiratory problems, colds and flu, warts and verrucas, burns and inflammation, fungal infections, cystitis, and sunburn. It can also be used undiluted on facial spots or insect bites.

• • • • •

Ylang ylang is a calming and relaxing oil that is good for easing stress. It is also noted for its aphrodisiac properties. It is widely used in skin care products to balance sebum secretion in the skin.

• • • • •

For an excellent skin tonic, make rosewater by mixing 1 tablespoon of rose oil with 4 pints (2.2 liters) of purified water. Bottle and store in the refrigerator.

• • • • •

Refresh combination skin by mixing two parts of rosewater with one part of witch hazel and apply to the skin with cotton balls.

• • • • •

For dry skin, combine 2 tablespoons lemon juice, 1 tablespoon glycerin, and 3 tablespoons rosewater, and rub into the skin.

• • • • •

For oily skin, dissolve 1 teaspoon borax in ¼ pint (150 milliliters) rosewater. Warm 2 tablespoons olive oil and slowly add to the mixture, then beat with an egg whisk until it is thick and creamy. Add 2 tablespoons lavender water.

• • • • •

For massage oil, mix ½ cup almond oil, ½ cup castor oil, and 1 teaspoon camphor oil together and shake well. Use after a bath or shower to soften skin and relieve tension.

. . . .

For sunburn oil, whip 1 tablespoon each of olive oil and glycerin together. Add 2 drops eucalyptus oil and paint gently onto the burned skin.

. . . .

Plant oils such as evening primrose, carrot, apricot kernels, or jojoba can be mixed with a little crushed pineapple and used as a mask.

. . . .

To soften the skin and relieve tension, take ½ cup almond oil, ½ cup castor oil, and 1 teaspoon camphor oil, and shake to mix thoroughly. Use to massage the body after a bath.

. . . .

As a skin moisturizer, warm 1½ tablespoons almond oil and 1 tablespoon lanolin in a dish over hot water. Add the contents of a vitamin E capsule and 2 teaspoons cold water. Smooth this preparation over the face and neck.

. . . .

For a natural odor repellent, combine ¼ cup vodka, 2 tablespoons witch hazel, 10 drops lavender oil, 1 drop juniper oil, and 1 drop lemon oil in a sterilized pump-lid bottle and shake before use.

. . . .

To remove make-up, coat the fingers with almond, sunflower, or avocado oil and spread evenly over the face and neck. Remove the oil with tissues.

· · · ·

To make a natural moisturizer for men, combine 2 teaspoons beeswax, 2 teaspoons lanolin, 2 tablespoons olive oil, 6 tablespoons infusion of thyme, and 12 drops cedarwood essential oil. Combine all the ingredients and use as required.

· · · ·

For blackheads, heat 4 tablespoons honey and add 1 teaspoon wheat germ, pat over the face, and leave on for 10 minutes. Wash off with warm water. Rinse with an astringent lotion.

· · · ·

For older skin, mix 1 tablespoon honey with a few drops of fresh orange juice. Cover the whole face with the mixture and leave for 20 minutes. Rinse well with tepid water.

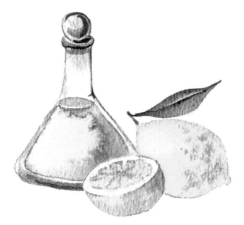

For problem skin, showing a minor outbreak of spots, mix 1 tablespoon honey with enough oatmeal to make a paste. Massage gently over the face and rinse well with tepid water.

. . . .

For flaky skin on the face, mix ¼ cup honey with ¼ teaspoon ground cloves and smooth on face. Leave on for 15 minutes, then rinse thoroughly.

. . . .

For an all over body scrub, mix 3 tablespoons finely ground oatmeal with 2 tablespoons almond oil. Scrub all over lightly, then rinse.

. . . .

For normal skin, make a mask by mixing a beaten egg white with ¼ teaspoon lemon juice or cider vinegar, or use a honey mask made with 2 tablespoons honey mixed with ½ teaspoon lemon juice or cider vinegar. When using these treatments, keep the hair tied back and don't go too close to the hairline.

. . . .

A honey and cream treatment is obtained by beating together 1 teaspoon honey with 2 tablespoons light cream. Leave on the face for 20 minutes.

. . . .

Mix 1 teaspoon honey with 2 tablespoons milk, and heat in the microwave for 15 seconds to melt the honey. Apply to the face, leave for 5–10 minutes, wash with warm water, then apply a moisturizer.

. . . .

Make an herbal pillow to give a soft fragrance to your bedroom and help you relax or induce sleep. The cover should be of thinly woven cotton and it is better to use dried ingredients for filling as the aroma lasts longer. Place the herbal pillow either inside or under you bed pillow.

· · · ·

For inducing sleep, mix lavender and thyme with a shake of cinnamon and dried grated orange peel.

Using Fruit & Vegetables

Avocado has a high vitamin content and is rich and nourishing for the skin. A dry or sensitive face, hands, or nails will benefit from a mask made from the pulp.

· · · ·

For normal to dry skin, mix some mashed avocado, tomato, strawberry, or banana with wheat germ or olive oil.

· · · ·

To soften skin, quickly mash 2 tablespoons avocado flesh with a few drops of lemon juice, to stop it going brown. Add 1 teaspoon honey and mix to a smooth paste. Apply to the face and leave for 20 minutes. Rinse off with warm water and then splash the face with rosewater. Towel dry.

· · · ·

For dry skin, leave the above avocado mixture on the face for 10–15 minutes while soaking in a hot bath.

· · · ·

For rough, dry skin on elbows, legs, or feet, rub the area with the skin of an avocado.

• • • •

A revitalizing mask for all skin types: mash ½ ripe, skinned avocado with 1 tablespoon tomato pulp and 1 tablespoon lemon juice. Smooth over the face and neck. Relax for 20 minutes and rinse off with tepid water.

• • • •

For dry skin, cut a piece of muslin to cover the face, and make holes for the eyes, nose, and mouth. Place over the face, then, using a pastry brush, apply mashed avocado or mayonnaise over the muslin. Leave the mixture on for 20 minutes, remove the muslin, tone, and moisturize.

• • • •

To help fade blemishes, mash a banana with 1 tablespoon of honey and leave on the face for 20 minutes. Wash off with tepid water. Or mash 1 large banana with 1 teaspoon each of fresh cream and milk. Add the oil from a vitamin E capsule and mix well. Apply to the face and neck and leave for 15–20 minutes. Remove with tepid water. Or rub a slice of melon over the face to freshen the skin. You can also make a face pack from a mashed slice of melon and half a peach. Smooth over the face and leave for 10 minutes. Rinse off with tepid water and pat the skin dry.

• • • •

For a skin toner, blend 1 peeled kiwi and 1½ teaspoons lime juice. Add an equal amount of water and blend until smooth. Use a cotton ball to apply to face. Refrigerate any leftover toner in an airtight container.

• • • •

As a skin freshener, wash, slice, and score the peel of three oranges and place in a saucepan with 3 pints (1.8 liters) of boiling water. Leave to steep until cold. Strain and use daily.

. . . . .

Mix dried orange peel with oatmeal paste and use as a face and body scrub. Use a slice of fresh pineapple to exfoliate dull or blemished skin.

. . . . .

For oily skin, mix equal amounts of white wine and lemon juice and dab over the skin. Or to make a facial scrub, add enough oatmeal to the wine and lemon to make a paste.

. . . . .

Or make a face mask by combining 2 teaspoons lemon juice, 1 teaspoon lime juice, and 1 teaspoon orange juice with 4 ounces plain unsweetened yogurt. Spread over the face and leave for 10 minutes. Rinse with warm water.

. . . . .

To remove excess hair on the face, mix 1 tablespoon fresh squeezed lemon juice with 4 teaspoons honey. Smooth on in the direction of your hair growth and leave on for 10–15 minutes. Rinse off. Use this mask twice a week.

. . . . .

As people age, tanned skin tends not to completely fade but it can look uneven. Mix the juice of 1 lemon, 1 lime, 2 tablespoons honey, and 60 milliliters plain yogurt. Gently massage into the skin once a week to lighten the skin tone and any age spots.

. . . . .

To get rid of rough, dry skin, grate the rind of one whole lemon into 4 tablespoons plain yogurt. Mix and rub over entire body concentrating on the driest patches. Rinse.

. . . .

To remove unwanted body hair, put ½ cup of lemon juice and 2 cups of sugar into a saucepan. Heat slowly until the sugar has melted. Boil rapidly for a few minutes until it becomes a caramel color, pour into a warm, sterilized jar and cool. Apply a layer of the mixture to the skin and smooth on a strip of linen, press down, then quickly pull the strip off going against the direction of the hair.

. . . .

Lemon juice is a time-proven freckle fighting remedy. Apply the juice with your fingers.

. . . .

To make body lotion for dry skin, combine 2 tablespoons lime juice with 3 tablespoons rosewater and 1 tablespoon glycerin until the mixture is smooth. Use after bathing.

. . . .

To make a cleanser for all skin types, mash 3 large strawberries with a fork, add ½ pint (300 milliliters) milk, and whisk well. Apply to the skin and leave to dry. Wash off with tepid water.

. . . .

For wrinkles, cut a grape in half and gently crush it on your face and neck. Leave for 20 minutes, then rinse off with tepid water and pat dry. Use daily.

. . . .

For sensitive skin or sunburn, mash two large strawberries with 1 tablespoon yogurt or cream. Smooth onto the face and leave for 10 minutes. Rinse off with tepid water.

• • • •

As a skin cleanser, mash 3 large strawberries to a pulp, add ½ pint (300 milliliters) of milk and whisk thoroughly. Apply to the skin and leave to dry. Suits all skin types.

• • • •

For dry or normal skin, make a paste with 2 teaspoons plain yogurt, 2 tablespoons raspberries, and 1 teaspoon fine oatmeal. Apply to the face and leave for 10 minutes. Rinse off with warm water.

• • • •

For a skin toner, rub mashed strawberries over the face after cleansing. Leave for 5 minutes, rinse off with tepid water, and moisturize.

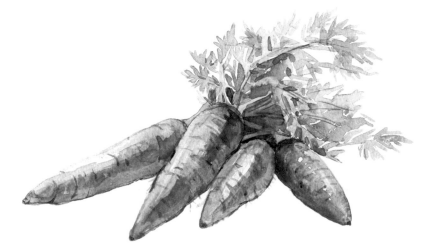

Rub a slice of raw tomato over the arms 2–3 times a day. Massage the juice into the skin with the palms of the hands. Let the juice dry on the skin and wash off with warm clean water to which a little borax has been added. Apply rosewater and glycerin mixed together. Blot off any excess with a tissue. This treatment will soften the skin.

. . . .

For a spotty back, blend 2 ripe tomatoes, add a carton of plain yogurt, and mix well. Smooth over the back and leave on for 20 minutes. Rinse off with tepid water.

. . . .

Juice a carrot and use as a mask for cleansing the skin. Use on all skin types; it is especially good for sensitive skin. For greasy skin, mix a little egg white with the carrot, or add 1 tablespoon mashed cucumber or tomato pulp to 1 tablespoon plain yogurt. Leave on the skin for 10–15 minutes and wash off with warm water. Pat dry.

. . . .

For a cleansing and soothing solution for all skin types, pour 7 tablespoons boiling water over 3 tablespoons finely chopped spinach leaves and 3 tablespoons grated carrot, cover, and infuse for 8 hours. Add ⅓ pint (200 milliliters), whisk, and infuse for 2 hours. Strain, bottle, and refrigerate.

. . . .

For normal or combination skin, exfoliate by rubbing with a potato cut in half. Use potato water as a cleanser for oily or blemished skin.

. . . .

Grate 2 inches (5 centimeters) peeled cucumber, and mix with 1 egg white. Spread the mixture over the face and leave for 15 minutes. Rinse off with warm water. Pat the skin dry with a towel.

·   ·   ·   ·

For a deep-cleansing mask, place 1 cup oats and 1 tablespoon wheat bran in blender. Grind to a fine powder. Add 1½ tablespoons lemon juice, 2 tablespoons buttermilk, 2 tablespoons whipping cream, 1 tablespoon plain yogurt, 1 teaspoon fresh mint leaves, and ½ medium cucumber, grated. Mix to a smooth consistency. Apply to just-cleansed face and leave for 10–15 minutes, then rinse off with warm water.

·   ·   ·   ·

Make a face mask by blending together ½ cup chopped cucumber, ½ cup chopped avocado, 1 egg white, and 2 teaspoons powdered milk. Apply 2 tablespoons as a mask to the face and neck in upward circular motions. Leave for 30 minutes, rinse with warm water, then a cold water rinse. Pat dry.

·   ·   ·   ·

Use slices of cucumber to soothe puffy or tired eyes. Pat mashed cucumber over sunburned skin.

·   ·   ·   ·

Blend up ½ cucumber and strain into a saucepan. Heat until simmering, bottle, and keep chilled. Use as a toner for all types of skin.

·   ·   ·   ·

Blend up a green pepper and add to any of your favorite face masks as nourishment for the skin.

·   ·   ·   ·

"An ounce of prevention is worth a pound of cure."
—Benjamin Franklin

Garlic has antiseptic qualities so it makes a good mask for blemishes. Beat 1 egg white to a froth, add 1 clove crushed garlic, 1 teaspoon kaolin, 1 teaspoon honey, and 1 teaspoon carrot juice. Use as a face mask. The slight smell of garlic will quickly evaporate.

· · · ·

Take a handful of lettuce leaves and cover with boiling water. Cool, strain, and use the liquid as a skin toner.

· · · ·

For a conditioning lotion, wash 8 lettuce leaves, cook in ½ pint (300 milliliters) milk for a few minutes until soft but still whole. Strain off the excess liquid and reserve. Lay the warm leaves on the clean face and press down gently. Relax for 20 minutes, then peel off the leaves. Rinse the skin with the strained milk.

· · · ·

Mix 2 teaspoons ginger with 2 teaspoons dried mustard, and add to bath. This is excellent for menstrual bloating and discomfort.

USING EGGS & DAIRY PRODUCTS

To make a face mask, beat the white of an egg until stiff and fold in 1 tablespoon of yogurt. Optional extras: Add 1 teaspoon honey for dry skin or 1 teaspoon lemon juice for combination skin. Leave on for 10–15 minutes, then rinse off with warm water.

· · · ·

For blemishes, blend 1 tablespoon of oatmeal with enough milk to make a paste. Add a whole egg (or a leftover yolk of egg) and mix well. Leave on face for 10–15 minutes and rinse first with warm water, then cool.

. . . .

For dry skin, combine 4 ounces plain yogurt with 2 tablespoons honey or combine a beaten egg yolk with 1 teaspoon honey and 1 teaspoon olive oil. Smooth over the face after a bath and leave for 5 minutes. Remove with cold water.

. . . .

For normal skin, mix 1 tablespoon honey and 1 tablespoon fresh cream. Smooth over the face and leave for 20 minutes. Rinse with tepid water.

. . . .

For oily skin, beat 1 egg white with 1 tablespoon honey until frothy. Smooth over the face and leave for 5 minutes. Rinse off with tepid water.

. . . .

For oily skin, blend up 2 ounces (50 grams) peeled, chopped cucumber. Add 2 teaspoons powdered milk and 1 whisked egg white.

. . . .

Or apply masks of various combinations using yogurt, egg white, or Fuller's earth mixed with lemon juice, cider vinegar, carrot juice, or mashed cucumber.

. . . .

For older skin, use slightly whisked egg white on its own or add 1 tablespoon powdered milk and ½ teaspoon honey. Beat well together until blended and brush onto the face. Allow to dry for 20 minutes before rinsing with tepid water.

. . . . .

To refine open pores, use beaten egg white, buttermilk, pulped tomato, cornmeal, oatmeal, bran, lemon juice, cider vinegar, and water, milk, or honey. Any of these ingredients can be used alone or mixed with any of the others. Make dry substances into a paste with a tepid liquid before applying.

. . . . .

Sensitive skin masks should be plain and simple. Use a couple of tablespoons of plain yogurt or mashed banana. Leave on for 5 minutes and only apply to the areas in need, such as a dry forehead or spotty chin.

. . . . .

For freckles, wash the face with sour milk. Lactic acid will provide a gentle peeling effect without irritating or drying skin. Or use a sour cream mask. Do not rinse this mask off completely, just remove gently with a facial tissue then apply a moisturizer.

. . . . .

To exfoliate skin gently, mix 3 teaspoons fine oatmeal with 3 teaspoons heavy cream, apply to skin, rub lightly and rinse off.

. . . . .

Warm 1 cup of milk in the microwave for thirty seconds (or until warm, but comfortable to the touch). Soak the hands for 5 minutes to strengthen nails and hydrate skin.

. . . .

For a bath soak, beat 2 eggs together with 6 tablespoons each of olive oil and sunflower oil, and 1 teaspoon honey. Continue beating hard and add 3 teaspoons mild shampoo, 6 tablespoons milk, and 3 tablespoons vodka. Finally add a few drops of favorite perfume oil. Add a dash of the mixture to a warm bath and relax.

. . . .

Add 2 pints (1 liter) whole milk and 3 tablespoons lemon juice, to a very warm bath. Slice the lemon and put in the water too. After 15 minutes you will be energized and your skin will be silky smooth.

. . . .

For normal skin, add 3 ounces (75 grams) ground almonds to ¼ pint (150 milliliters) milk and mix well. Simmer until the liquid is absorbed and add a beaten egg yolk. Reheat until boiling and add 1 tablespoon almond oil. Cool and use to massage the body before bathing.

. . . .

For greasy skin, mix an egg white with an equal amount of lemon juice and half a cup of water. Spread over the skin and rinse off after five minutes.

. . . .

Close pores with a skin-tightening all-natural clay or mud mask, or mix 1 egg white with a few drops of lemon juice. Using a brush, massage onto clean skin. Leave on for 5 minutes, then rinse with warm water.

. . . .

For a detox bath, add 1 pound (500 grams) baking soda and 8 ounces (225 grams) sea salt to warm water. Soak until water is cool.

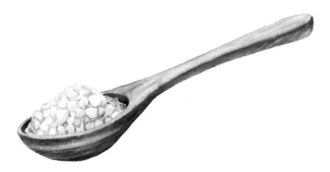

Healthy Habits

DID YOU KNOW?

Sugar ages skin as much as smoking or excessive sunbathing.

. . . .

Foods you crave and eat the most may be causing most of your health problems.

. . . .

Nearly 45 miles of nerves run through our bodies.

. . . .

The average human body contains 600 muscles.

. . . .

Half the body's red blood cells are replaced every seven days.

. . . .

The skin accounts for 12 percent of the body weight.

. . . .

Thirty-one pairs of spinal nerves originate from the spinal cord.

. . . .

During a lifetime, the kidneys clean over 1,000,000 gallons of blood.

. . . .

As the body develops, the heart grows at the same rate as your fist.

. . . .

Half a liter of water is lost every day through breathing.

. . . .

Women's breasts are really modified sweat glands.

. . . .

The surface area of the lungs is about the same size as a tennis court. The left lung is smaller than the right lung to make room for the heart.

. . . .

The small intestine is nearly twenty feet (six meters) long.

. . . .

Babies have more taste buds than adults but prefer bland food.

. . . .

An average human body contains 40 liters of water.

. . . .

80 percent of all of the body heat escapes through the head.

. . . .

The liver is the body's largest organ, weighing 3–5 pounds in adults.

. . . .

The average human produces 2 pints saliva a day or 10,000 gallons in a lifetime.

. . . .

Messages travel along the nerves as electrical impulses at speeds up to 248 mph.

SLEEP TIGHT

There are many theories on how much sleep we need. Lying awake worrying that we are not getting enough sleep only intensifies the problem.

. . . .

A guideline of sleep requirement is, if you feel drowsy during the day, or if you fall asleep within five minutes of sitting down, you are not getting enough sleep.

. . . .

Infants require about 16 hours sleep a day while teenagers need 9 and adults 7–8 hours.

. . . .

Regular exercise daily promotes better sleep. A few hours before bedtime get some fresh air or go for a short walk.

. . . .

Some people find it can upset their biological clock if they do not have a regular routine of going to bed and getting up at set times.

. . . .

Rise earlier in the morning and you will be tired at bedtime.

. . . .

About an hour before you want to go to bed, start winding down. Read a book, write a letter, or listen to music rather than watching a gripping show.

. . . .

"A good laugh and a long sleep are the best cures in the doctor's book."
—Irish Proverb

If soft music helps you relax, many radio alarms are set to switch off automatically after an hour, so you have no worry about the radio being on all night.

. . . .

A warm bath is always relaxing; try adding a few drops of lavender or marjoram oil.

. . . .

Make sure you have a comfortable mattress.
To avoid becoming preoccupied with your inability to sleep, try counting backwards from 100, or go through the alphabet and find a different thing you like for each letter.

. . . .

Think of how you would spend a windfall of ten thousand dollars!

. . . .

Do not eat a heavy meal before going to bed; a warm milky drink will make you feel sleepy.

. . . .

Soft drinks, coffee, or alcohol should not be taken late at night as they increase the activity of the mind.

. . . .

If you find that you have some problem or something you want to remember the following day, have a notepad and pencil at your bedside and write it down.

. . . .

Keep the bedroom pleasantly warm but not stuffy. Heavy window curtains will stop the dawn light from waking you.

. . . .

If you cannot get to sleep, then get up and rest. Rather than forcing yourself to sleep go and lie down on a sofa or comfortable chair, close your eyes, and try to relax. Stay there until you feel really sleepy.

. . . .

To relieve tension in the upper body, sit cross-legged and block the ears with your fingers. Breathe in, then breathe out making a humming sound, to lengthen the exhalation. Repeat 10 times before going to bed.

. . . .

In bed, try consciously relaxing each part of your body in turn, slowly working up from your toes.

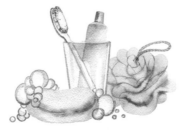

"Nothing cures insomnia like the knowledge that it's time to get up."
—Unknown

There are five stages of sleep patterns we go through:
- **Stage 1:** a light sleep where we drift in and out and can be woken easily. Muscle activity starts to slow.
- **Stage 2:** eye movements stop and the brain waves become slower with some bursts of rapid waves.
- **Stage 3:** very slow brain waves or delta waves start to develop, in a deep sleep.
- **Stage 4:** brain only produces delta waves. Will be in a deep sleep, difficult to wake. There is no eye movement or muscle activity and if woken will feel disorientated.
- **Stage 5:** REM or rapid eye movement sleep. The eyes jerk rapidly, the breathing is more rapid and irregular, the heart rate increases, and limb muscles become temporarily paralyzed. This is when dreaming occurs and REM sleep stimulates the brain regions used in learning.

• • • •

For chronic insomniacs, research has developed a method that is quite successful. You must have a week free to allow you to sleep during the day. The idea is to alter the body's natural sleep rhythm from its later sleep pattern to an earlier one, bringing it back to normal. The sleep rhythm is found to be more easily altered by extending the waking day. For example, if you are not going to sleep normally until 4–5 a.m., the first night, you would stay awake until 7:30 a.m. The second night, stay awake until 11 a.m. Continue extending your bedtime to 2 p.m., 5 p.m., and 8 p.m., ending up going to bed at 11 p.m. on the sixth day. Keep going to bed at 11 p.m. and you should find your sleep pattern should be settled by this time.

STRESS CONTROL

Excessive stress and tension can affect your health, so keep them under control.

. . . .

Avoid working more than 10 hours a day. Take at least one day off from the normal work routine every week, to spend at leisure. Rise 15–20 minutes earlier and enjoy the morning.

. . . .

If a work schedule for the day is an extra long list, don't panic. Select what is urgent and deal with them first. The rest can be done if you have time or kept for another day.

. . . .

Take some time for yourself every day. Know how you are going to spend this break so that you don't waste the time wondering what to do or scrolling through your social media feed. Read a book or start some craft work. Plan and enjoy every minute of your break.

. . . .

Concentrate on the present. Stop dwelling on the past or worrying about the future.

. . . .

Learn to say no. Too many favors or too much volunteer work can leave you without any free time.

. . . .

"Remember it takes a long time to grow an old friend."
—Unknown

Don't compete with your friends, neighbors, or coworkers. Be your own person and live your life accordingly.

. . . .

Be realistic and avoid setting unattainable goals that will only cause frustration if you cannot achieve them. Try not to be a perfectionist in everything—no one is perfect.

. . . .

Exercise at least three times a week. In addition to sports, walking, jogging, running, and going to the gym, remember that things like gardening or chopping wood are excellent ways to relieve tension.

. . . .

"Smile and the whole world smiles with you." Be pleasant to people around you. Words of appreciation to others will make you feel good.

. . . .

Have fun, laughter, and a good sense of humor. Take a look at yourself and think of all your good points. When you're dealing with other people, look out for their good points. Avoid always being critical and negative.

. . . .

There's pleasure in giving as well as receiving, so enjoy doing kind deeds.

. . . .

Stop being obstinate and learn to give in. There is generally a way around most things rather than straight through.

. . . .

Learn to express your feelings and emotions openly, without unnecessary aggression.

. . . .

Sometimes it helps to write down the things that annoy you, how you would solve the problem, and how you feel about the situation. This can be a first step in relieving stress.

. . . .

"A problem shared is a problem halved" is very true. Find someone you feel you can trust—it may be a religious leader, a therapist, or a relative or friend. Talk over your problems and perhaps a different approach could solve your worries.

. . . .

Drink at least 8 glasses of water a day. Eat a healthy diet (high fiber, low fat food) and have your meals at regular intervals. Reduce your caffeine and sugary foods intake.

. . . .

Tension from stress can interfere with the muscles of the intestines. To restore normal movement in the gut, bend the knees, place hands on the thighs, and keep the back straight. Exhale sharply and poke the stomach out. Keeping the lungs empty, quickly contract and expand the stomach muscles 9 times.

. . . .

Learn to breathe properly to slow the heart rate, lower blood pressure, and reduce stress levels. Correct breathing through the nose 16 times a minute is beneficial to all the body. First place the forefinger and the middle finger of the left hand on the bridge of the nose. Breathe out through both nostrils. Put the thumb over the side of the left nostril to close it and inhale through the right nostril. Close the right nostril with the fourth finger, lift the thumb of the left nostril and breathe out. Pause. Then leaving the finger in place, inhale through the left nostril. Close the left nostril with the thumb and breathe out through the right one. Repeat the exercise 5 times. This should be done daily to reduce shallow breathing.

· · · ·

Drugs used to control stress can become addictive very quickly. They may relieve the obvious symptoms but do nothing to change your behavior or way of life. Alcohol and cigarettes do not relieve stress, and sometimes they exacerbate it.

· · · ·

Learn relaxation techniques and practice them daily. When you feel under pressure and tense, close your eyes and count back from 20, saying each number silently on the out breath.

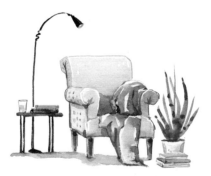

Watch out for jaw, neck, and shoulder tension; learn to consciously relax these areas.

· · · ·

Close your eyes and imagine a square. Breathe out to a count of 2 as you travel along each side. Repeat 3 times.

· · · ·

Sit down and close your eyes. Breathe in and out for 5 minutes, holding the out-breath twice as long as the in.

· · · ·

When things are really getting to you, sometimes the best solution is to have a good scream. Open your mouth wide and scream. Shout out any angry words or thoughts. If you do not want to be overheard, then howl into a pillow or cushion.

· · · ·

Try to have at least one vacation away from your work and home environment every year. Be careful not to turn the self-catering holiday into work.

· · · ·

Relaxation allows the mind to drift into a pleasant dream-like state while meditation is a state of relaxed alertness that helps to tune out from the endless stream of mental chatter.

· · · ·

Try to meditate at the same time and place every day. The place should be comfortable, warm, well-ventilated, and pleasing to the senses.

· · · ·

Since lying down is generally the sleeping position, it is not recommended for meditation. Instead, try these positions:
- Sitting on the floor cross-legged.
- Sitting on the floor against a wall with the cushion placed in the small of the back, legs outstretched, and feet together, hands resting on the thighs.
- Sitting in a straight-backed chair with the feet flat on the floor and hands resting on your lap.

· · · ·

Close your eyes and empty the lungs by breathing out through the mouth with a sigh. Breathe in through the nose, allowing the abdomen to extend and sink slightly as you breathe in and out.

· · · ·

Starting at the feet and moving to every part of the body in turn, until you reach the scalp, think relaxation. Be aware of your breathing, but breathe naturally, making no effort to control it. Become aware of the still-point between the in-breath and the out-breath. On every out-breath count 1, then 2, up to 10. Count only once on the out breath and when 10 is reached go back to 1 again. Keep counting for 10 minutes.

· · · ·

To return to normality, imagine you are centered along a straight line running from the top of the head to the feet. Open the eyes, shake out all the limbs, and have a good stretch. Get up slowly.

SOCIAL DRINKING

Although an irregular party binge of alcohol will not do any
lasting damage, it can make you feel very ill the following
morning or day. Try to avoid this situation.

. . . .

It takes the body an hour to metabolize 1 unit of alcohol. This
is equivalent to a 350-milliliter bottle of beer with 4.5% alcohol,
a glass of wine, or a measure of spirit in a mixer. Drinking 2–3
drinks in an hour is more intoxicating than sipping those same
drinks over the course of an evening.

. . . .

Generally, the higher the concentration of alcohol, the more
quickly alcohol is absorbed. Spirits are around 40% alcohol, so
they are absorbed faster than beer, which averages 3–5% alcohol.

. . . .

Carbonated drinks like champagne are absorbed faster than non-
carbonated drinks, like wine.

. . . .

Given equal amounts of alcohol consumed in 1 hour, remember
that women get drunk more quickly than men, due to the
relativity of body weight. Older people generally achieve higher
blood alcohol levels than younger people.

. . . .

It can take 20 hours after your last drink for all the alcohol to be
eliminated from the body. It is impossible to speed up this process.

. . . .

"Many things can be preserved in alcohol. Dignity is not one of them."
—*Unknown*

Although drinking a glass of milk before "partying" may help,
it is very important to have a good meal beforehand. High fiber
foods like pasta or whole grain bread will help absorption.

· · · ·

Drink clear drinks like white wine or white spirits as red drinks
tend to give hangovers. Never mix drinks made from grapes
(wine) with drinks made from grain (whiskey).

· · · ·

If drinks are served with a slice of lemon, transfer it to each new
drink; a glance will show how many drinks have been consumed.

· · · ·

Alternate mineral water or fruit juice with alcoholic drinks. Or
have 2–3 alcoholic drinks and then change to soft drinks.

· · · ·

Mind your glass so that no one can add more alcohol without you
noticing. Do not keep "topping up" your glass as you will lose
track of how many drinks you've had.

· · · ·

If you don't feel like drinking but people are harassing you, use
the excuse that you are driving, or on antibiotics.

· · · ·

Drink a few glasses of water before you go to bed, as dehydration is the greatest cause of hangovers.

. . . .

Do not give a person coffee to sober them up as it is a diuretic; it depletes fluid and makes alcohol in the body even more concentrated.

. . . .

If, however, you do wake up with a hangover and the two main symptoms are headache and thirst, then the only cure is time and rest. It takes the liver 1 hour to filter 1 unit (a glass of wine, a shot of spirits, or half a lager), but it will take another few hours to recover.

. . . .

Do not be tempted to have another drink. It only raises the blood alcohol and it is a very dangerous habit.

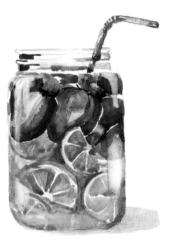

Drink plenty of water or orange juice. Eat honey. Salty foods will replace lost sodium and thus make you thirsty. Avoid spicy or acidic foods. When you do feel able, it does help to eat a nourishing meal.

• • • •

Alcohol absorbs vitamin B, so replenish this with plenty of nuts and fruit.

• • • •

Alkali products may calm your queasy stomach.

• • • •

To speed up the detoxifying process, eat a bowl of plain yogurt with a chopped banana and a spoonful of honey added. Drink a glass of fruit juice.

Non-Toxic Cleaning Solutions

TREATING FABRIC STAINS

Try to treat stains immediately. If you have no available removal remedy, soak the article in cold water.

· · · ·

If this does not work, try lukewarm water with ordinary soap or scented soap. Dampen the fabric and rub with soap until the stain is erased. Rinse with lukewarm water, put between two towels, and pat until damp dry. Do not use hot water as this can set the stain.

· · · ·

If the stained material is colored, always test the removal remedy on an inconspicuous area first. After applying the removal remedy, rinse the fabric thoroughly in plenty of lukewarm water. Then wash as usual.

· · · ·

When working on a stain, always work in towards the center as working outwards will spread the damage.

· · · ·

To avoid watermarks, place the wet article on a towel and press another towel on top.

· · · ·

To whiten woolen garments that have yellowed, mix one part hydrogen peroxide with eight parts water and soak the garment in this for 12 hours.

· · · ·

"We never know the worth of water 'til the well is dry."
—English proverb

Yellowed cottons or linens can be brightened by boiling the items for one hour in 1 gallon (3.8 liters) of water with 1 tablespoon (15 milliliters) each of salt and baking soda added.

. . . .

Whites that have yellowed from over-bleaching can be restored by soaking in warm water with 2 tablespoons (30 milliliters) malt vinegar added.

. . . .

Wine stains—apply table salt to a wet wine stain immediately. Allow the salt to absorb the wine. Rinse off with cool water. Reapply if necessary.

. . . .

Beer stains—immediately sponge with a mild vinegar solution. Rinse with lukewarm water, apply a paste of wet biological washing powder, leave for 30 minutes.

. . . .

Old beer stains can be difficult to remove. Soak the garment in cold water overnight and proceed as above.

. . . .

Remove ink stains from washable clothes by spraying with hairspray or perfume, then press between absorbent paper. Or soak ink stains immediately in milk.

. . . .

Dried ink stains: rub with a cut tomato and wash well.

. . . .

To remove beet stains from clothes, rub half a cut pear over the mark.

. . . .

Remove wash-in hair color on a towel by spraying with hairspray.

. . . .

Lipstick stains on clothing can be removed by rubbing with a piece of stale bread. On washable material, soak in vinegar and water.

. . . .

Orange juice or tomato stains—sponge with a mixture of ¼ ounce (6 grams) borax in 1 pint (600 milliliters) tepid water.

. . . .

Black currant or blackberry stains—if still wet can be rubbed with lemon juice. If the stain has dried, then soak in glycerin and wash in hot water.

. . . .

Soot—never rub soot from fabric; cover the area with salt, then brush with a stiff brush.

. . . .

Tar stains—to remove from unwashable material, make a paste of powdered Fuller's earth and turpentine. Rub in well around the stain. Leave to dry and then brush off with a clean stiff brush.

. . . .

Remove tar or oil stains from white socks by rubbing with toothpaste.

. . . . .

On washable material, rub the tarred area with lard, butter, or salad oil. Scrape off any loose tar after a few hours.

. . . . .

Fresh blood stains—on washable clothes, immediately soak in cold water. Rub with soap and cold water, rinse well. Add a few drops of ammonia or hydrogen peroxide to the water if the stain is resistant.

. . . . .

Dried blood—soak the stains overnight in biological washing powder and cold water or in 1 gallon (3.8 liters) water with 8 ounces (200 grams) salt added.

. . . . .

Stubborn bloodstains—mix liquid dish soap with milk and apply to the stain.

. . . . .

On unwashable fabric such as blankets, use a paste of raw starch and lukewarm water. Spread on the stain and, when paste is discolored, brush off with a soft brush.

. . . . .

Grass stains—on jeans or pants, treat by rubbing gently with lemon juice before washing. On other material, dampen the stain with cold water, apply cream of tartar, and leave for a few hours.

. . . . .

"The man who removes a mountain begins by removing small stones."
—Unknown

Tea and coffee stains—to remove from white tea towels, soak in water with a dissolved denture cleaning tablet. Sugar sprinkled over a fresh tea stain will make it easier to wash out.

. . . .

Bicycle oil—to remove from pants, massage the stain with liquid dish soap.

. . . .

Bicycle grease, suntan lotion, and gravy stains—use scented soap to remove stains from clothes.

. . . .

Dirty shirt collars—rub shampoo into the collars, leave for ten minutes, then wash as usual. Or apply a paste of vinegar and baking soda and leave for 15 minutes.

. . . .

Cooking oil or grease—dab on some talcum powder over the marks before washing.

. . . .

Urine stains—sponge with a solution of baking soda and water to neutralize the acid and remove the smell.

. . . .

Perspiration stains—soak garments in water with a dash of white vinegar or a handful of baking soda. Which method will work on your clothes depends on your body chemistry. Or dissolve a couple of crushed aspirin tablets in the washing water.

LAUNDRY

Before hanging out clothes in cold weather, wet your hands with vinegar and rub in until dry. This will prevent your hands from chapping.

. . . .

Rubbing cornstarch on your hands will help prevent your skin from cracking in the cold, dry air.

. . . .

Reduce excess soap suds in the washing machine by adding a dash of vinegar or lemon juice with half a cup of water to the powder compartment—the suds will disappear.

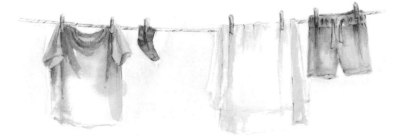

Before using new towels, soak them in cold water overnight and then wash as normal.

. . . .

To stop jeans from fading, before the first wash, make a solution of 7 ounces (220 grams) salt to a bucket of warm water and soak the jeans for 24 hours. Then wash as normal. Or soak for 30 minutes in 1 gallon (3.8 liters) water with 4 tablespoons (60 milliliters) added vinegar.

. . . .

Add starch to the rinsing water when washing nylon tights or stockings to help prevent runs and snags.

. . . .

Wash silk gently by hand in a warm, soapy water solution. Rinse thoroughly, adding 4 tablespoons (60 milliliters) white vinegar to 1 gallon (3.8 liters) water for the final rinse. Iron while still damp.

. . . .

Wash mohair or lambswool garments with a mild hair shampoo, then add a little hair conditioner to the final rinse.

. . . .

Add 1 tablespoon (15 milliliters) sugar to hand-washing water and you will find that it helps to remove grime.

. . . .

Stop color running into the white parts of multi-colored clothes by adding 1 tablespoon (15 milliliters) salt to the washing powder.

CLEANING HINTS

An all-purpose cleaner for painted walls: Wear rubber gloves and mix 1 cup (250 milliliters) ammonia, ½ cup (125 milliliters) vinegar, and ¼ cup (62.5 milliliters) baking soda with 1 gallon (3.8 liters) warm water. Wash thoroughly and rinse.

. . . . .

Soften old chamois leather cloths by rinsing them in 4 pints (2.5 liters) of water with 1 teaspoon (5 milliliters) of olive oil added.

. . . . .

Urine odors on a mattress may be neutralized by dampening the spot and sprinkling with borax. Rub the borax into the area and let dry. Brush or vacuum to remove the dry borax. Pet urine and sour milk odors can be neutralized using the same process.

. . . . .

Remove pet hairs from fabric by putting on a pair of thick household rubber gloves and rubbing your hands over the surface of chairs, carpets, etc.

. . . . .

Clean leather bags by rubbing them with the inside of a banana skin or with a cloth dipped in egg white and whisked until frothy. Polish with a soft cloth.

. . . . .

Revive shabby suede shoes by sponging with vinegar. Stuff with newspaper and leave to dry. Rub lightly with sand paper and then with a stiff brush.

. . . . .

"What most of us need most is to need less."
—Unknown

Buff polished leather shoes with an old pair of tights.

FLOOR COVERINGS

Use water from boiled potatoes to freshen discolored carpets.
This also helps to remove mud stains from carpets. Rinse with
clean water.

. . . .

To restore and brighten carpet colors, sprinkle a mixture of tea
leaves and salt over the whole carpet, then vacuum or brush off.

. . . .

Make your own carpet cleaner by adding 2 tablespoons
(30 milliliters) each of salt and white vinegar to a bowl of warm
soapy water.

. . . .

For a wine stain on a carpet, soak up the excess as quickly as
possible. Cover the stain with an absorbent powder such as salt
or talcum powder. When the powder becomes sticky, remove
it and add more until most of the stain has gone. Apply a final
layer of powder and leave for two hours, then brush this off.
Any remaining marks can be removed by rubbing with a cloth
dampened in a mild detergent solution. Rinse with a clean wet
cloth, rub dry, and air well.

. . . .

"It is the neglect of timely repair that makes rebuilding necessary."
—Richard Whately

Burn marks on carpets: Slight marks caused by sparks can be removed by rubbing vigorously with the cut surface of a raw onion or a raw potato.

· · · ·

Remove stains from darker carpets by rubbing with used coffee grounds. Brush in well, allow to dry, then vacuum as usual.

· · · ·

Dried coffee stains: Remove from a carpet by rubbing a few drops of glycerin into the mark to loosen it, then leave for a few hours. Squeeze out a cloth in warm water with a little liquid dish soap added, and wipe the area.

· · · ·

Table salt will absorb spilled ink. Pour salt on the wet ink and continue to add salt until there is no more wet ink. Then vacuum or wash.

· · · ·

Milk stains: Mix six parts water, two parts ammonia and a pinch of salt, dampen a soft cloth with this solution, and use to remove the stains.

· · · ·

Fresh coffee stains: Remove with saltwater.

· · · ·

Lambskin rugs: Brush with plenty of dry powdered magnesia. Leave for a day, shake well, and brush thoroughly.

• • • •

Clean the brushes on the vacuum cleaner with a dog's metal comb.

• • • •

Ballpoint pen ink can be removed from vinyl by rubbing with a slice of raw potato.

• • • •

To clean linoleum: Wear household gloves and make a solution of ½ cup (125 milliliters) of household bleach and a ¼ cup (62.5 milliliters) each of white vinegar and washing soda. Add this to 1 gallon (3.8 liters) warm water. Use the solution to mop your linoleum floor.

• • • •

To brighten old linoleum, mix one part of fresh milk with one part turpentine. Rub the mixture onto the floor and polish with a warmed soft cloth.

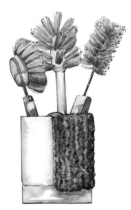

To clean floor and wall tiles, dissolve 4 ounces (100 grams) of shredded coarse soap and 4 ounces (100 grams) washing soda in 1 gallon (3.8 liters) hot water. Scrub the tiles with the solution and a stiff brush. Rinse and dry.

WOOD

Black streaks on banister rails or tops of chairs can be removed by mixing equal drops of turpentine and vinegar with enough powdered laundry starch to make a paste. Carefully rub the area with the mixture. Rinse off with warm water.

. . . . .

To clean a wood block floor, rub lightly with a fine steel wool pad moistened with turpentine substitute. Rub with the grain. As the polish and grime softens the dirt, wipe it off. Re-polish when dry.

. . . . .

Black heel marks on light-colored floors can be removed with white spirit or turpentine.

. . . . .

Pen marks on wood, plastic, or other hard surfaces can be removed by using cotton balls dipped in aftershave.

. . . . .

Clean varnished woodwork or floors with cold tea. Then polish with a soft duster.

. . . . .

To remove slight water marks on polished wood, rub with a cloth dipped in metal polish, then use wax polish to shine.

. . . . .

To remove large water marks on polished wood, rub with an equal mixture of linseed oil and turpentine substitute.

. . . .

White ring marks on tables from wet or hot dishes or glasses can be removed by rubbing a thin paste of vegetable oil and salt on the spot with your fingers. Leave for a couple of hours then wipe it off.

. . . .

Use lavender furniture polish on woodwork for a fresh smell and to discourage flies.

. . . .

To avoid getting metal polish on stained wood when cleaning a mail slot on a door, wipe the wood around the brass with paper towel dipped in cooking oil. After polishing, wipe off the oil with clean paper.

. . . .

To remove paper stuck on wood, moisten with baby oil and leave for a few minutes; it will peel off easily.

. . . .

To clean cork table placemats, put them in a bowl of clean cold water and rub each one gently with a pumice stone. Rinse under cold running water. Dry in a cool place. Do not use soap or warm water.

CLEANING CONCOCTIONS

Be sure to store all cleaning solutions out of reach of young children and pets.

• • • •

Carpet cleaner: Dissolve 2 ounces (50 grams) of yellow washing soap in 2 pints (1.2 liters) boiling water, then add ½ ounce (2.5 grams) washing soda and 3 tablespoons (45 milliliters) ammonia. Mix thoroughly and pour into carefully labeled jars. Mix 2 tablespoons (30 milliliters) of the mixture in 2 pints (1.2 liters) warm water and rub onto the carpet with a brush or cloth. Rinse off with a clean water and cloth. Dry well with a dry cloth. Open the windows and doors to air the carpet. Do not saturate the carpet or the backing will rot.

• • • •

Non-slip sheen for wooden floors: mix equal parts of paraffin oil and vinegar in a screw top plastic jar, shake well, and apply sparingly to the floor with a dry cloth. Repeat monthly.

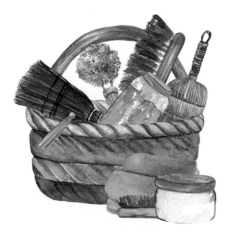

"To scrub a floor has alleviated many a broken heart."
—Unknown

Make a polishing cloth: Mix 3 tablespoons (45 milliliters) each of paraffin (or linseed) oil and vinegar in a screw top jar. Put a duster into the jar to absorb the liquid. Then hang out to dry. Use to polish furniture and store in the jar when not in use.

· · · ·

Silver dip: Half fill a 32-ounce jar with silver paper (chocolate bar wrappers are best). Add 2 tablespoons (30 milliliters) table salt and fill the jar with cold water. Cover the jar and keep near the kitchen sink. Dip stained silver silverware in the mixture and leave for two minutes to remove any stains. Rinse thoroughly.

· · · ·

Brass polish: Mix ½ teaspoon (2.5 milliliters) salt and ½ cup (125 milliliters) white vinegar with enough plain flour to make a paste. Apply the polish to the brass and leave for half an hour. Rub and wipe off with clean cloth.

· · · ·

Chrome polish: Use apple cider vinegar. Wet a cloth with the vinegar, wipe on the chrome. Dry with a clean towel.

· · · ·

Copper polish: Mix together lemon juice and salt. Apply to the copper and scrub with scouring pad.

METALS

Silver: Use pieces of raw rhubarb for cleaning silver. Or place silver in potato cooking water until it shines.

. . . .

Tarnished silver articles: Add 1 teaspoon (5 milliliters) baking soda and 1 teaspoon (5 milliliters) salt to 1 pint (600 milliliters) of almost boiling water. Immerse silver in it and leave until tarnish has disappeared. Rinse in warm water and dry with a soft cloth. Or crumple some tin foil and place it in a bowl of water. Put the silver in the water and let it soak for a couple of hours.

. . . .

Tarnished silver with intricate patterns: Clean using toothpaste on a soft toothbrush.

. . . .

Dull gold jewelry: To bring instant shine, rub with a cut tomato. Rinse well.

. . . .

Pewter: Clean by rubbing with the pithy side of a piece of orange or cabbage leaves. Polish with a soft cloth.

. . . .

Rusty or tarnished brass curtain hooks: Soak them in ammonia, then boil in the water in which haricot beans have been cooked.

. . . .

Neglected brass will clean easier if it is first washed in a solution of strong ammonia. Or leave the article in a cola drink overnight.

. . . .

Brass ornaments: clean using a dash of cider on a cloth.

. . . .

Dirty brass and copper: Bring back the shine by rubbing with half a lemon dipped in salt. Wash well in soapy water and rinse thoroughly before giving a good buff.

. . . .

When using store-bought brass cleaner, add some lemon juice for better results.

. . . .

A soft cloth dipped in white spirit makes an economical cleaner for brass.

. . . .

Polish brass with a soft cloth and a few drops of olive oil. Rinse off with water and liquid dish soap. Finally, polish with a clean cloth.

. . . .

After polishing brass, give it a quick rub with flour for a longer lasting shine. Or spray with hair lacquer. Protect any surrounding wooden area with newspaper first.

. . . .

Lacquered or varnished brass should never be scoured. Instead, apply a paste of lemon juice and cream of tartar. Leave for five minutes and then wash with warm water and dry thoroughly with a soft cloth.

. . . .

Tobacco stains: clean stains from brass or nickel ashtrays by applying alcohol with an old toothbrush and then washing in hot vinegar and salt.

. . . .

Bronze: To clean bronze, dust well and rub the surface with a little warmed linseed oil. Polish with a chamois leather. Avoid using water or white spirits on bronze.

. . . .

Chrome: Rub with a damp cloth and dry starch or baking soda. Rinse, dry thoroughly, and polish well.

. . . .

Stainless steel faucets, etc.: Rub occasionally with a cloth dipped in paraffin to keep them gleaming.

. . . .

Rusted iron or steel: Soak in paraffin for one to two days to soften the rust. Gently rub the wet surface with emery paper.

GLASS

To remove fly spots from electric bulbs, dampen soft paper towel in a mixture of equal amounts of vinegar and water, then rub this over the bulbs.

. . . .

Rub the inside of fish tanks with salt to remove hard water deposits, then rinse well before returning the fish to the tank. Use only plain, not iodized, salt.

. . . .

Another window cleaning solution: Mix 3 tablespoons (45 milliliters) white vinegar with 4 pints (2.5 liters) water. Apply with a clean cloth. Dry off with a chamois leather or a crumpled sheet of newspaper.

· · · · ·

Crumple old newspaper into a ball and slightly dampen it, then use to clean windows. Polish off with crumpled dry newspaper.

· · · · ·

To reduce condensation on windows in cold weather, place a cup of salt on the windowsill to absorb the room's moisture. Or rub a little glycerin over the inside of windows once a week.

· · · · ·

Rub lavender essential oil over windows and frames to keep flies out of the kitchen.

· · · · ·

Wash windows at a shady time of day. Wear sunglasses when cleaning windows and you'll see the smears more easily.

· · · · ·

After washing outside windowsills, spray them with furniture polish and they will stay cleaner for longer.

· · · · ·

When stacking delicate glass bowls on top of each other, put a folded piece of paper towel in the bottom of each dish. This avoids breakage and keeps the bowls from sticking together.

· · · · ·

"Criticism is the disapproval of people not for having faults, but for having faults that are different from your own."
—Unknown

To make inexpensive glassware sparkle, rub a paste of baking soda and water on the glass. Rinse under cold running water. Dry and polish with a soft cloth.

. . . .

Rub down a small chip on the rim of a precious wine glass with emery paper to smooth it.

. . . .

Keep cut glass and crystal vases clean by lining with a clear plastic bag before each use.

. . . .

To clean a badly stained, narrow necked vase, tear up newspaper and place in the vase. Fill with warm water. Leave overnight and shake the paper around, then empty the vase and rinse well. Or put a strong salt solution in the vase and shake, then wash the vase with soap and water. Or clean with a solution of a proprietary brand of toilet cleaner diluted in a little water. Leave for an hour and rinse well before use.

. . . .

If a stopper is jammed in the neck of a decanter, put a few drops of cooking oil or glycerin around the rim and leave overnight. Tapping the stopper gently with the back of a wooden brush will often remove it.

. . . .

To clean a decanter or carafe, fill with warm water and 1 tablespoon (15 milliliters) baking soda. Add some crushed eggshells or rice grains. Leave for several hours, shaking regularly. Rinse with hot water and dry in the sun. Or use a solution of equal amounts of warm water and vinegar with half a cup of sand. Shake well and leave overnight. Rinse well.

· · · · ·

Lime stains caused by hard water can be removed in the same way as above but use tea leaves with the vinegar.

· · · · ·

To remove wine stains from a decanter, add chopped raw potato and warm water, shake vigorously for a few minutes. Or add a little ammonia to the washing water and scrub with a brush. Rinse well.

GENERAL CLEANING

Tapestry: Sprinkle with powdered magnesia and work it in well with a clean cloth held between your fingertips. Leave overnight or for several hours, then brush out gently with a soft clean brush.

· · · · ·

Remove marks from old china and porcelain by painting with neat bleach, or rub brown marks with a damp cloth dipped in salt until they disappear.

· · · · ·

"It's better to lose sleep on what you plan to do than to be kept awake by what you have done."
—Unknown

To clean the inside of a clock, soak a small piece of a cotton ball in kerosene or paraffin and place in the base of the clock. Leave for a few days. This will draw down all the dust and leave the clock clean.

. . . .

Ivory piano keys: Clean with a little toothpaste on a damp cloth. Use milk to rinse. Polish off with a soft cloth. Or rub with a cloth sprinkled with hydrogen peroxide or pure lemon juice. Never use water on ivory. If possible, leave keys exposed to sunlight as they yellow in the dark. Sprinkle French chalk between the keys to prevent them from sticking.

. . . .

Gilt picture frames: Mix one egg white with 1 teaspoon (5 milliliters) baking soda. Sponge the surface with the mixture. Or use a little dry cleaning fluid on a cloth.

. . . .

Plaster statuettes: To remove dirt and grease, mix a paste of finely powdered starch and hot water. Apply the hot paste with a brush. Leave to dry; the starch will absorb the grime and flake off.

. . . .

Leather furniture: To prevent it from drying out, mix two parts raw linseed oil with one part wine vinegar. Shake well and apply evenly with a soft cloth, then polish.

. . . .

Use a broad clean paintbrush to dust the tops and fronts of books stacked on a shelf.

. . . .

Marble: Clean by painting the surface with a mixture of one part powdered pumice, one part powdered chalk, and two parts baking soda. Leave on for a day and wash off with clean water and a soft brush. Or wash with a strong solution of saltwater with an added dash of vinegar.

. . . .

To remove green algae from a headstone, wash with a solution of one part hydrogen peroxide to three parts water, plus a few drops of ammonia. Rinse well with water.

. . . .

Oil stains from a concrete driveway: remove by pouring a little cola drink over them to dissolve the mark.

. . . .

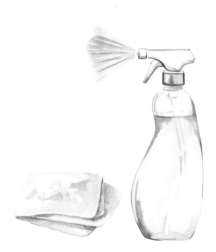

Grease or oil on concrete: Clean by putting kitty litter over the stain. Leave to soak up the grease, then sweep up. Alternatively, shake dry laundry detergent on the grease, dampen the powder, and leave to absorb the grease. Wash off with water.

. . . .

Concrete stained with black coloration from the weather is usually mold. Spray a solution of one part bleach to three parts water on the concrete. Brush in and leave for a few hours. Wash off with clean water.

Index